HueTrition®

Fun & Simple Nutrition for the Whole Family

MONICA H. SAN MIGUEL

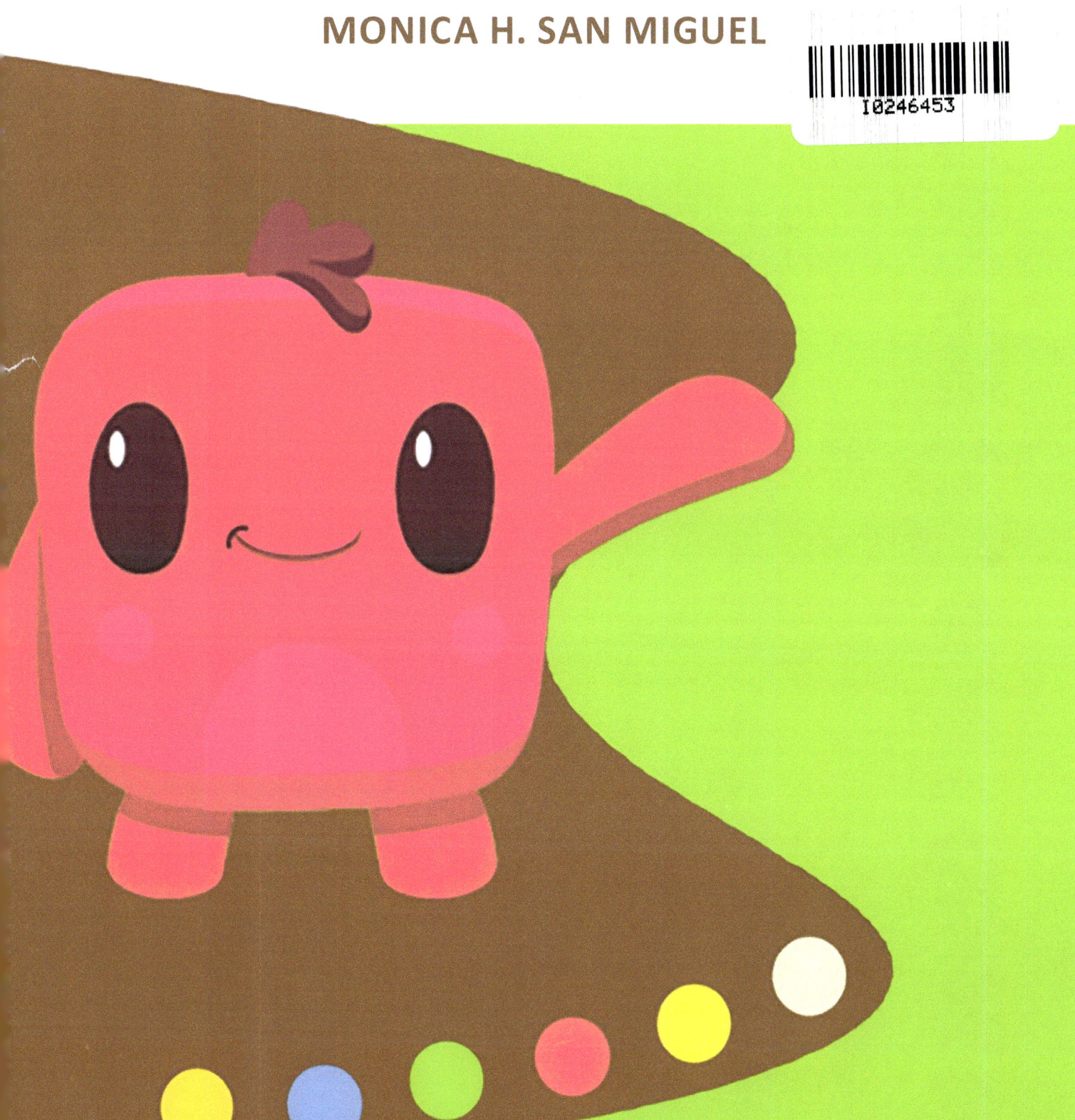

Our Story

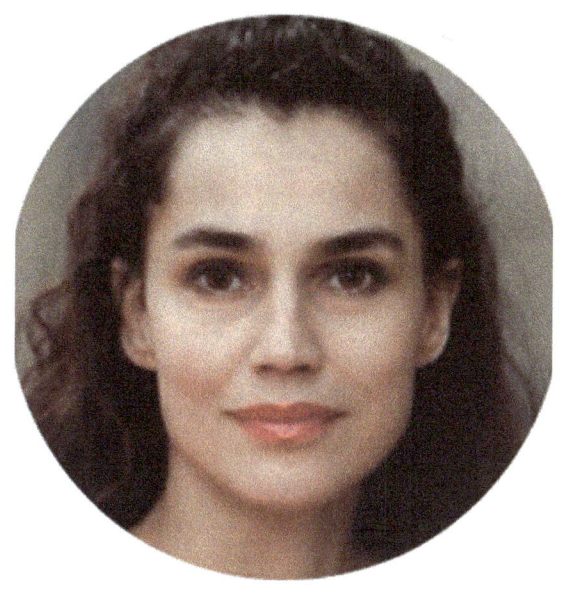

Monica H. San Miguel, CEO & Founder of HueTrition, is a food and health industry visionary, digital innovator, and author. She is passionate about nutrition and driven in her desire to spread the word about healthy eating. Having spent more than 18 years in a variety of leadership roles in the food, health and wellness industries, she is uniquely qualified for the job!

A life-long athlete, played tennis at both the collegiate and professional levels, earning a full athletic scholarship to Texas A&M University.

She is the proud mother of two children, and an entrepreneur with a mission to create a HueMovement to encourage kids and families to lead a healthy, colorful lifestyle.

Why I created HueTrition?

To make nutrition Simple and Fun with Color.

Our simple philosophy, Food is Fuel to Color Your World. Natural, colorful, sustainable, filling half of your plate with fruits and vegetables solves a lot of problems. Think of your plate as a colorful canvas.

How is HueTrition different? It is the simplest and most fun way to eat healthier.

HuePets is a mobile app that turns daily healthy eating into a game. The opp is tied to a website that allows you, family, and friends to view your dashboard of colorful choices and even assign rewards!

We have created a list of HueApproved products, brands, restaurant dishes that you can view at HueTrition.com

Our simple criteria for HueApproved:

o Real food
o As wholesome as possible
o Pronounceable & fewer ingredients
o Color packed- fuel to color your world

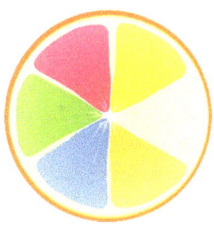

Creating healthier families, one smile at a time.

HueTrition™ is a nationally-recognized family wellness program that utilizes cutting-edge technologies to promote a balanced, active, lifestyle that includes a daily variety of colorful fruits and vegetables from an early age while encouraging sensible choices for the planet.

- Help school professionals, dietitians, educators, and parents encourage a healthier lifestyle in children from an early age
- Free technology-based tools for parents and educators, including games and activities that make nutrition fun
- Promoted across HueApproved ™ brands, products, schools, restaurants, retail/grocery, and social media channels
- Supported by leading dietitians and medical professionals

HueMovement™: a multidisciplinary coalition of like-minded brands and organizations that support a plant-based colorful lifestyle

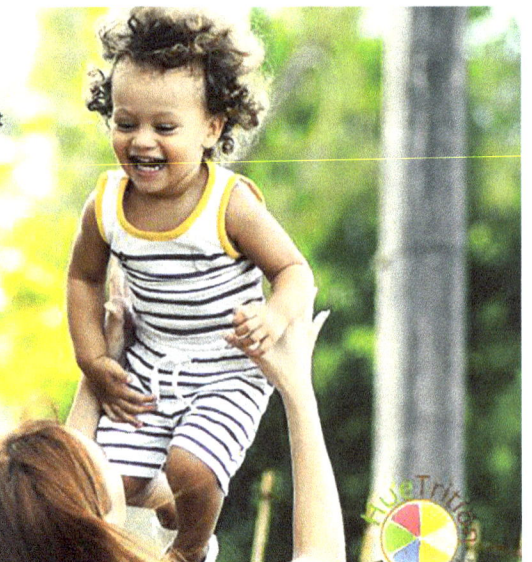

HueTrition is a lifestyle that focuses on eating a daily variety of health promoting, pure colored and minimally processed foods, namely fruits and vegetables. Embracing HueTrition is about fostering a permanent, positive change through incorporating a whole spectrum of fruits and vegetables into your diet ("you are what you eat, right?").

HueTrition is NOT a diet, but if you have been struggling to lose weight or simply would like to shift towards a plant-based lifestyle, you will begin to substitute your snacks and side dishes with colorful vegetables. During this time, you will not only begin to notice improvements in your energy levels and weight, but more importantly, you will be on your way to fool-proofing yourself against chronic disease (coupled with regular physical activity of course!).

info@HueTrition.com
HueTrition.com

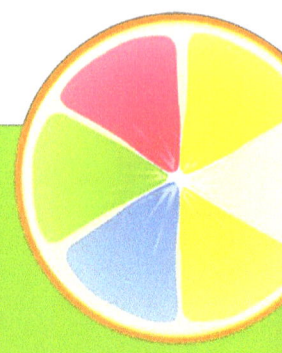

Did you know the color of fruits or vegetables can tell you the vitamins and nutrients they have?

We recommend at HueTrition.com to aim for one of each of the 5 colors every day. At HueTrition we divide these foods into 5 categories, by color: blue/purple, red, green, yellow/orange, and white. Dividing fruits and vegetables by color provides an easy way to incorporate nutrient needs and health benefits into our diet.

Eating by color is easy

As you read through the chapters and pages of this book, you will find that it really is as simple as eating by color to get the nutrients your body craves and needs for health.

The second half of this book is a children's book

This book also serves as a guide to children. You will find the second half of the book is a story you can read to your children, one that invites them into the world of choosing food through color. We also encourage you to check, HuePets, a fun way to encourage them to eat fruits and vegetables – a mobile app that turns healthy eating into a game. It is important to get kids excited about eating fruits and vegetables, because the choices they make at a young age can shape choices for the rest of a child's life.
For more information, please visit HuePets.com.

You can download the HuePets app at the AppStore or Google Play

Recipes for you to make with your children and family

Five recipes are included for you to make for your family, as well as five recipes for your child and you to make together. You can find more tips and recipes by visiting our website: HueTrition.com

Color makes food look appetizing

Food companies also use a rainbow of colors, because people are attracted to colors in their food. Very often it is not the food that contains these colors, though. It is merely the wrapper or box holding the food, meant to be appetizing or attractive. There is a reason why candies are dyed bright colors.

info@HueTrition.com

HueTrition.com

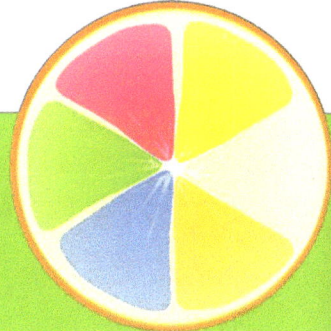

We eat with our eyes and bright colors appeal to the appetite. Plus, without all the packaging, fruits and vegetables are better for the environment!

Freshness and nutrient value of a fruit or vegetable by the richness of its color

When you walk through a produce section, you can quickly tell the quality or freshness of a fruit or vegetable by its color. These colors are also telling us something else. They are telling us how nutrient-dense our food is. Fresh foods and colorful foods are our best choice, our best diet, and our best medicine.

Nature has made something easy for us to understand. So easy, in fact, that even a child can understand. Now, let's read on.

A child's palate adjusts to diet

When your child is eating healthy, their palate is conditioned to perceive sweetness in sweet fruits and vegetables. When a child is eating a lot of sugar, they may not perceive the sweet fruits and vegetables as being sweet because they might be conditioned to the very strong sweetness of sugar.

Consider this: A friend posted a photo of her 9-month old baby online eating his first bite of ice cream-- blue cotton candy ice cream. What did the baby do? Wince and spit it out.

On my niece's first birthday she had cupcakes, and what was her response to her first encounter with the sugary food? *A grimace.*

These children had so far only had baby food, and purees of fruits and vegetables. To them, those pureed yams were very sweet. And they still can be, for both you and your child. What we would like to do is preserve this sense in our children, of really tasting the sweetness in natural foods. Our palate, or sense of taste, is conditioned by our diet.

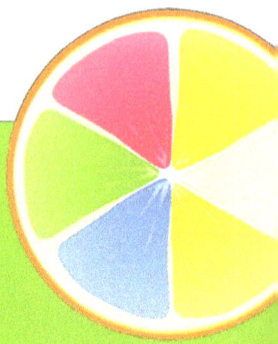

info@HueTrition.com

HueTrition.com

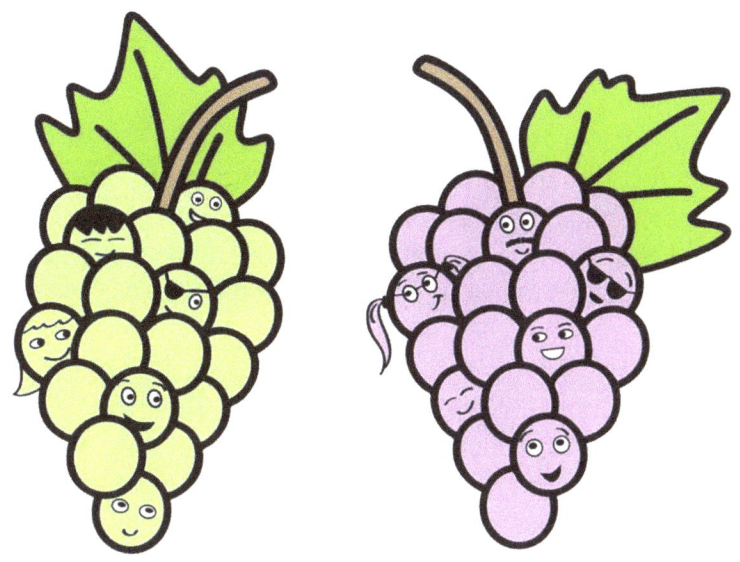

WHATEVER COLOR, YOU CAN ALWAYS FIND A BUNCH!

CHAPTER 1
Blue and Purple Fruits and Vegetables

Blueberries, plums- fresh and dried (prunes), blackberries, eggplant, purple grapes and raisins, purple Belgian endive, purple asparagus, black currants, purple carrots, elderberries, purple figs, purple peppers, purple/blue potatoes, purple corn

These blue and purple foods are high in antioxidant flavonoids, specifically anthocyanins. Anthocyanins protect cells from damage. They may reduce cancer and stroke risk, and heart disease. Purple and blue foods are also high in phenols, antioxidants that may prevent heart disease and bolster the immune system.

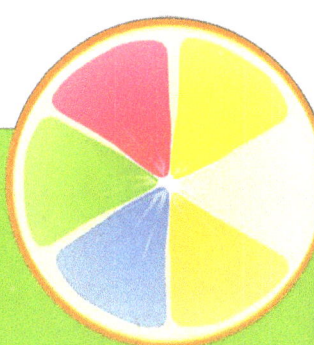

info@HueTrition.com
HueTrition.com

Some of the more common blue fruits and vegetables are expanded upon below:

Blueberries

Blueberries are often considered a nutritional powerhouse in a teeny tiny package because they have the highest antioxidant level of any fruits. Blueberries are also a good source of Vitamins A, C, E and beta-carotene as well as rich in the minerals potassium, manganese, and magnesium. The antioxidants come in the form of anthocyanins.

Plums or dried prunes

Plums and prunes help in the production and absorption of iron. Plums have a high content of vitamin C. Plums and prunes are high in a unique antioxidant called neochlorogenic or chlorogenic acid. Plums are good for the eyes and prevent macular degeneration. Plums also have anticancer properties.

Blackberries

Blackberries are rich in Vitamin A and Vitamin C. They are a good source of potassium and contain calcium, B vitamins, zinc, copper, and magnesium.

Eggplant

Eggplant has low levels of vitamins and nutrients, but it has high levels of the antioxidant phenolic acid. One of the most potent phenolic compounds contained in eggplant is called chlorogenic acid, which is one of the strongest eliminators of free radicals that can damage cells in the body. Other benefits of chlorogenic acid can include antimicrobial, anti-bad cholesterol, and anti-viral activities.

Purple Grapes (sometimes referred to as black grapes)

Resveratrol is found in purple grapes, bilberries, blueberries and cranberries. It is concentrated in the skins, and in those fruits that have seeds, in the seeds as well. It is anti-cancer, anti-viral, neuroprotective, anti-aging, and anti-inflammatory. This compound is also found in red wine made from purple or red grapes. Like red grapes, they also contain vitamins C, B-1, and B-6. They also contain quercetin in the skin. Quercetin is a strong antioxidant that can fight free radicals. It decreases the effects of aging, and guard the body from disease. Quercetin is also found in pears, apples, onions and citrus fruits. Antioxidant properties of grapes can

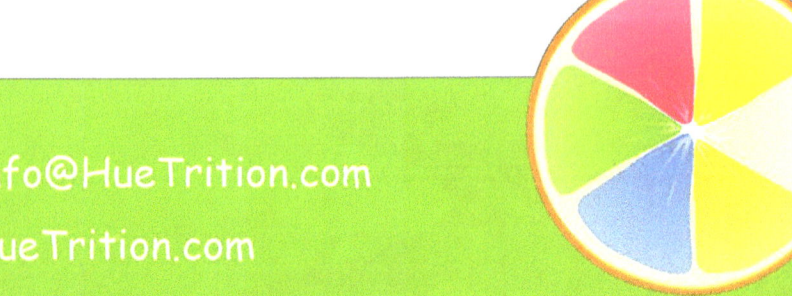

also be attributed to their phenol content. The phenolic content of grapes in the form of anthocyanins also contributes to the color of the grapes.

Raisins

Raisins are a great source of iron and potassium. Did you know that raisins contain a phytonutrient called oleanolic acid that destroys the bacteria that causes cavities? Raisins are one of the best sources of boron, a mineral that aids in bone health. Black raisins contain the phytochemical resveratrol. Resveratrol reduces stroke risk and is an antioxidant, is anti-inflammatory and anti-cancer, and can even lower blood cholesterol.

Easy Ways to Incorporate Blue Fruits and Vegetables Into Your Diet

- Add a handful of blueberries to oatmeal, yogurt, or pancakes.

- Have a small glass of grape juice.

- Pack grapes for a snack or with lunch.

- Make hors d'oeuvres by stuffing purple Belgian endives with avocado or anything creamy. Endives are delightfully light and crunchy, great paired with something creamy.

- Snack on raisins or prunes. Dried fruits are handy to keep around. They're chewy, have a concentrated sweet flavor, and a long shelf life in your cupboard.

- Find a great eggplant recipe, such as Eggplant Parmesan.

- Shop the farmers market if you are looking for some of the more unusual foods, such as purple carrots or asparagus and blue potatoes.

- Freeze berries-and this works for many other fruits- so that they will last longer and can then be used for smoothies.

info@HueTrition.com
HueTrition.com

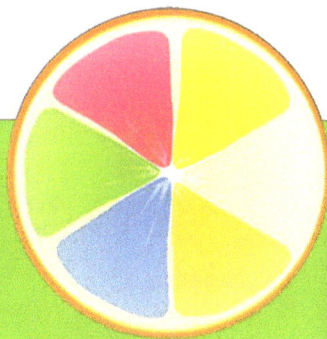

Test your Blue/Purple HQ with these 5 questions:

1.) Are anthocyanins antioxidants?

2.) Are anthocyanins flavonoids?

3.) Are flavonoids antioxidants?

4.) What antioxidant does eggplant have a lot of?

5.) What two antioxidants are contained in the skin of purple grapes?

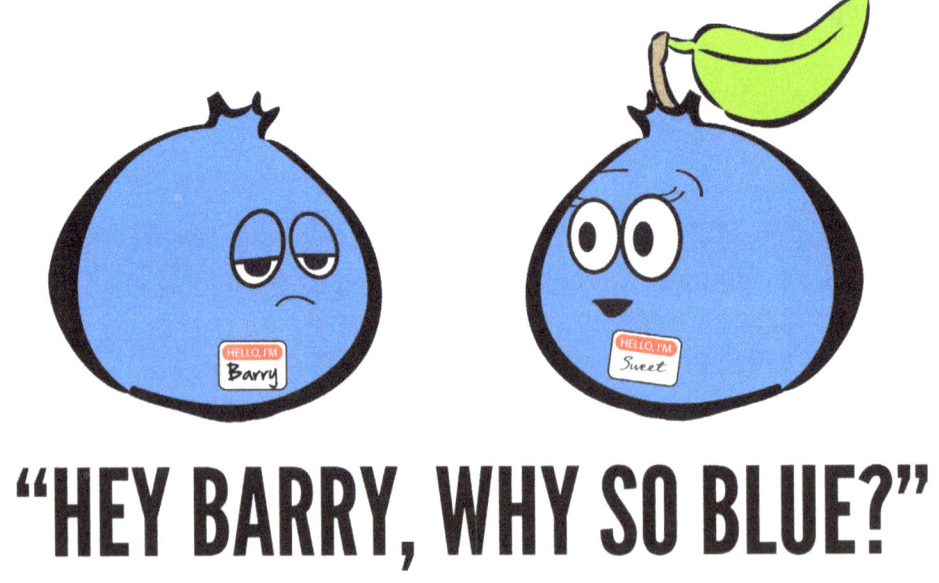

"HEY BARRY, WHY SO BLUE?"

info@HueTrition.com

HueTrition.com

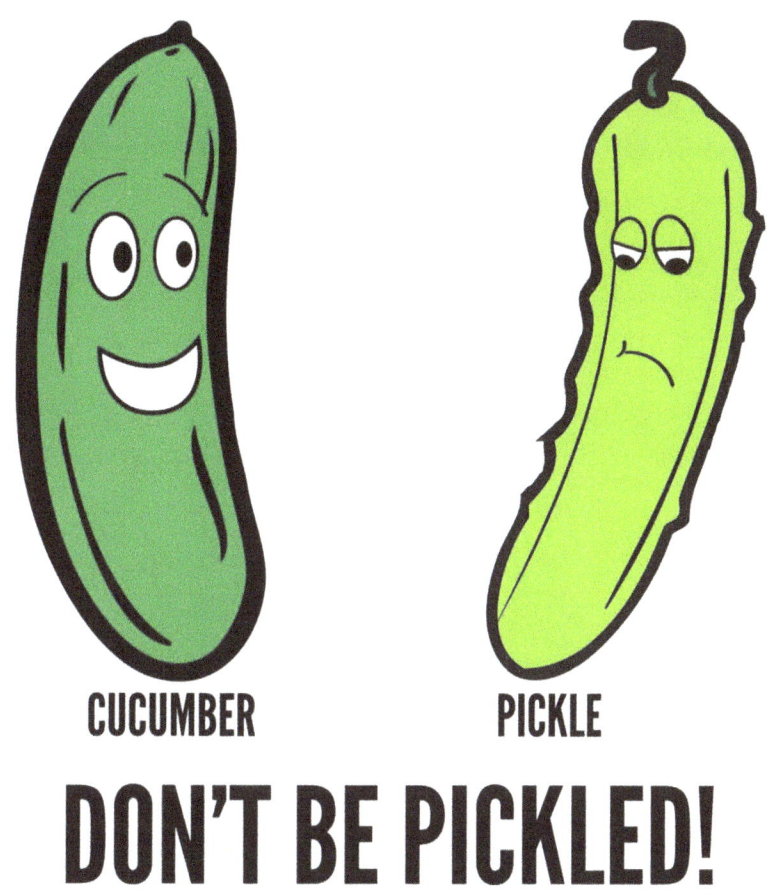

CUCUMBER   PICKLE

DON'T BE PICKLED!

CHAPTER 2
Green Fruits and Vegetables

Green vegetables are colored by chlorophyll, a natural plant color. Lutein found in chlorophyll works in conjunction with another chemical called zeaxanthin found in egg yolk, corn, red peppers and oranges. So don't be afraid to pair these in dishes, such as broccoli with red bell peppers or... better yet have an omelet that includes broccoli and red bell peppers in the filling, accompanied by a glass of orange juice.

Another thing many green vegetables have in common is that they have vitamin C to support our immune systems.

info@HueTrition.com
HueTrition.com

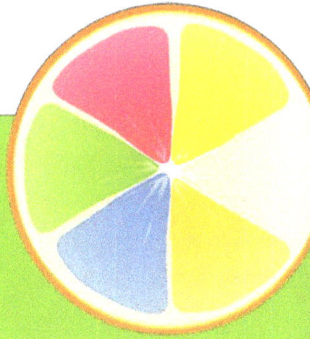

Green Vegetables-

Green peppers, zucchini, cucumbers, artichokes, asparagus, green beans, broccoli rabe, celery, chayote squash, Napa cabbage, bokchoy, endive, leeks, iceberg lettuce, okra, scallions, celery, artichokes

Dark green leafy vegetables-

Spinach, collard greens, kale, swiss chard, romaine lettuce, arugula, turnip greens, dandelion greens

Dark Leafy greens contain lutein, which keeps eyes healthy. These green vegetables are often dense in vitamin K.

Dark leafy greens such as spinach and kale are sources of B vitamins including folate, iron, and calcium. Dark green colored vegetables include more vitamin C than light green colored vegetables. Romaine lettuce has 8 times the beta-carotene and 6 times the Vitamin C of iceberg lettuce.

Cruciferous green vegetables- broccoli, brussel sprouts, green cabbage

The "indoles" found in cabbage, broccoli, brussel sprouts, and other cruciferous vegetables have been studied as possibly preventing cancer.

Green Fruits-

Kiwi fruit, honeydew melon, limes, peas, green beans, green grapes, avocadoes, green apples, and green pears

Some popular green fruits and their nutritional values are:

Kiwi fruit-

Kiwi has vitamin C and vitamin E and minerals such as potassium, magnesium and phosphorus. Eating kiwi may be good to reduce and protect against asthma symptoms, help reduce macular degeneration, its good for cardiovascular health.

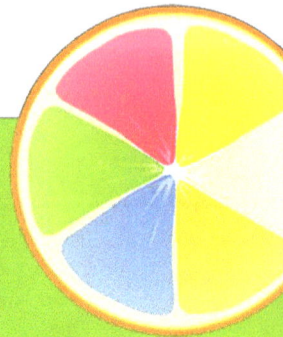

info@HueTrition.com
HueTrition.com

Honeydew melon-

Honeydew is a good source of potassium, Vitamin B6, folate, and Vitamin C.

Limes-

Citrus limonoids found in lime and other citrus fruit have been shown to fight cancers of the stomach, mouth, lung, skin, breasts and colon. Limes are a great source of Vitamin C, folic acid, potassium, vitamin B6 and flavonoids.

Peas-

Peas are a good source of protein, fiber, vitamins, minerals, and lutein. They are a good source of vitamins A, C, and Niacin and the minerals potassium, phosphorus, and magnesium. They are most dense in vitamin K, like green beans, and green grapes.

Green Beans-

Green beans contain high amounts of vitamin C and vitamin K, manganese, vitamin A, dietary fiber, potassium, folate, and iron.

Green Grapes-

Green grapes are high in vitamin C and vitamin K. Green grapes, like all grapes, are high in phytochemicals. Green grapes also contain calcium, iron, magnesium, phosphorus, potassium, zinc, copper, manganese and selenium, as well as vitamins A, B6 and thiamine, niacin, pantothenic acid, riboflavin and folate.

These are not categorized as vitamins or minerals but they have an active role in the body. Phytochemicals are lower in green grapes then in red varieties and do not contain resveratrol, a chemical found in those darker grape varieties.

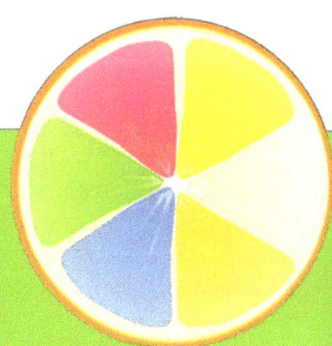

info@HueTrition.com
HueTrition.com

Avocadoes-

Vitamins in avocadoes include vitamin A, B vitamins, antioxidant vitamins C and E, and the minerals phosphorus and magnesium. They are low in sugar and starch and high in easily digestible fats. They make a great slow-burning fuel and are great to eat to keep your blood sugar stable, so you don't get energy highs and lows. Avocadoes contain fourteen minerals, including iron and copper.

Green apples such as Granny Smith-

Green apples have vitamin C and folate. Like most fruits and vegetables they are high in fiber, but what they also contain is pectin, a compound that binds to fat and flushes it from the body. Apples are rich in phytonutrients, organic compounds of plants that are beneficial to our health: quercitin, zeaxanthin and beta carotene. The quercitin is found in the skin of green and golden apples.

Quercetin is a flavonoid found in certain fruits and vegetables aids in the prevention of cancer, heart disease and other diseases. Quercitin, in the human body, has shown anti-inflammatory, anti- allergic, anti-microbial, and anti-cancer action. Evidently, quercetin and other flavonoids can change the body's reaction to viruses, allergens, and carcinogens. Quercetin has been explored as a treatment for certain cancers. An apple a day really does keep the doctor away!

Green pears-

Pears have a low glycemic index (G.I.). A low G.I. is good for everyone, diabetics included, because it means that the food digests slowly, and the glucose or sugars from the food are released slowly. Foods with a high G.I. release all their sugar very quickly into the blood stream, causing the pancreas to produce more insulin as well as a burst of energy that is not sustained. Foods with a high G.I. can lead to weight gain because the body does not have time to digest the sugars.

They are hypoallergenic- allergies and sensitivities to pears are rarely if ever found. They are good for pulmonary disease, cancer prevention, and inflammation. Green pears also quercetin in the skin. These phytonutrients have been found to be antioxidants that have anti-cancer and anti-inflammatory properties.

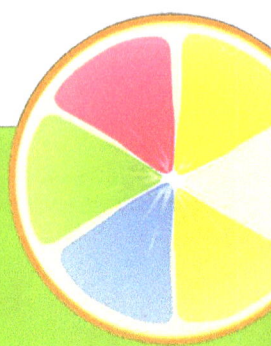

info@HueTrition.com
HueTrition.com

Easy Ways to Incorporate Green Fruits and Vegetables Into Your Diet

- Make eating green fruits delicious and fun for a child: Cut up and put green fruits on a skewer (a great way to incorporate other fruits as well) and dip into vanilla yogurt.

- For quick preparation, buy baby spinach. It is usually prewashed and sautés in just a few minutes.

- For a quick and colorful side, sauté some zucchini slices with cherry tomatoes in olive oil over medium heat, and towards the end add some Parmesan.

- Pack a green apple or pear for snack or for lunch. Top an apple with peanut butter for a great kids treat.

Test your Green HQ with these 3 questions:

1.) What gives green fruits and vegetables their color?

2.) What does G.I. stand for and what does it mean?

3.) What are phytochemicals or phytonutrients?

info@HueTrition.com
HueTrition.com

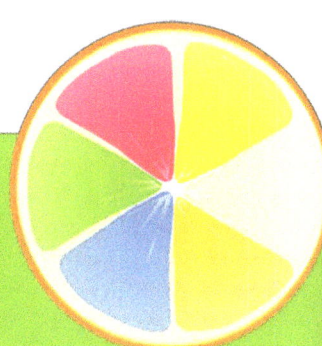

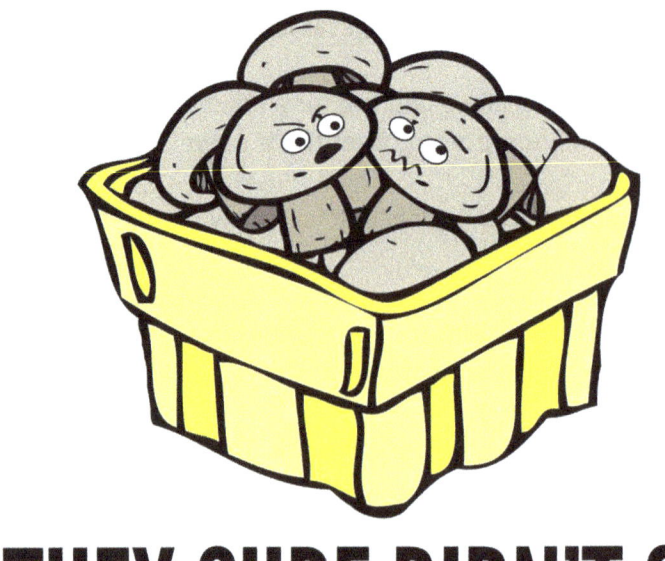

"THEY SURE DIDN'T GIVE US 'MUSH ROOM' IN HERE!"

CHAPTER 3
White Fruits and Vegetables

Allium Family- garlic, onion, shallots

Vegetables from the allium family such as onions and garlic are good for blood circulation and blood vessels. Mushrooms are known tumor fighter but they must be cooked first. Garlic is sometimes known as nature's antibiotic. Both onions and garlic are good for the common cold.

White vegetables

Mushrooms, cauliflower, ginger, jicama, parsnips, turnips, white potatoes, bamboo, hearts of palm, water chestnuts

info@HueTrition.com
HueTrition.com

White Fruits: banana, white peaches, brown pears

White fruits and vegetables are colored by natural plant pigments called "anthoxanthins."

These may help lower cholesterol and blood pressure. They also may reduce the risk of stomach cancer and heart disease.

Both bananas and potatoes are good sources of potassium.

White Potatoes

White potatoes provide 30% of your recommended daily amount of vitamin C, 2% of your recommended daily calcium, and 10% of your daily iron needs.

Easy Ways to Incorporate White Fruits and Vegetables into Your Diet

- Freeze a banana with a stick inserted for a frozen, creamy treat. Take it one step further and put the banana in the blender. It comes out smooth and creamy like ice cream.

- Garlic, onions, and shallots can all improve the savory flavor of any vegetable, soup, pasta or dish. In a little olive oil on low heat in a pan simply sweat the onion or shallot until it is translucent and softer, add some optional mushroom slices, then add the garlic for 30 seconds until it is fragrant, golden, but not burned. Sauté spinach or sauté blanched vegetables (vegetables that have been submerged in already boiling water until just tender and bright colored).

Test your White HQ with these 2 questions:

1.) What compound is responsible for the color of white foods?

2.) Bananas and potatoes are rich in what mineral?

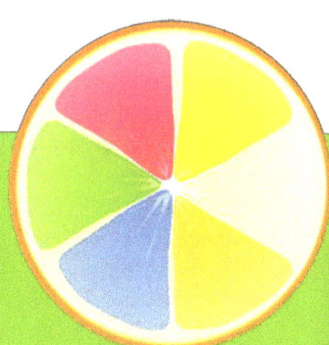

info@HueTrition.com
HueTrition.com

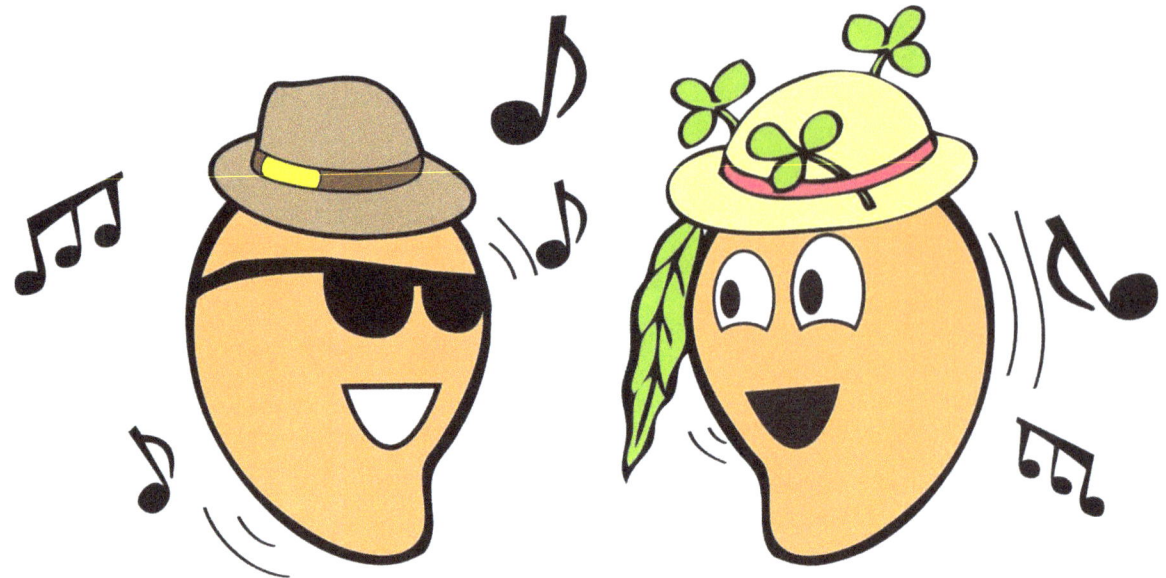

IT TAKES TWO... TO MANGO!

CHAPTER 4
Yellow/Orange Fruits and Vegetables

Yams, Carrots, Pumpkins, kobucha squash, acorn squash, acorn squash, yellow beets, butternut squash, carrots, yellow peppers, persimmons, yellow potatoes, rutabaga, sweet corn, yellow tomatoes, yellow winter squash, spaghetti squash

Yellow/Orange Fruits

Oranges, peaches, papayas, nectarines, mangos, apricots, cantaloupe, pineapple, yellow grapefruit, lemon, yellow apples, cantaloupe, yellow figs, golden kiwifruit, yellow pears, tangerines, yellow watermelon

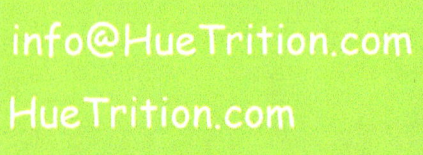

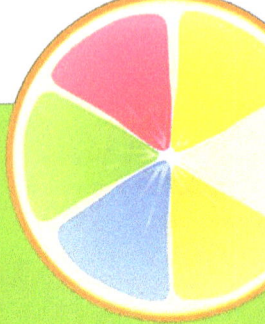

Beta-carotene

According to a 10-year study from the Netherlands about carrot consumption and cardiovascular disease (CVD) where foods with deeper shades of orange yellow were compared with green, red, purple, and white, foods with deep shades of orange/yellow were proven to be the most preventative against cardiovascular disease. The George Mateljan Foundation site, The Worlds Healthiest Foods, details this study in their article "The Latest News About Carrots" (http://whfoods.org/genpage.php?tname=btnews&dbid=164).

Beta-carotene is usually what gives orange fruits and vegetables their color. Yellow and orange fruits and vegetables are usually colored with naturally occurring plant colors called "carotenoids." Beta-carotene gets converted into Vitamin A, it is good for the eyes, and can improve heart health, protect from cancer, and build a healthy immune system.

Carotenoids

Carotenoids are great for eye health. One study found that people who ate a high-carotenoid diet were 43% less likely to get macular degeneration, an eye disorder common among older people.

Some commonly eaten orange/ yellow fruits and vegetables in detail:

Carrots

Carrots are known for their high beta-carotene content.

Oranges

Oranges are a great source of Vitamin C and the B vitamin folic acid.

Sweet Potatoes

Sweet Potatoes provide more nutrients than red or white potatoes. One medium sweet potato contains 120% of the recommended vitamin A, 30 percent of the total vitamin C, and 4% or the recommended allowance for calcium and iron.

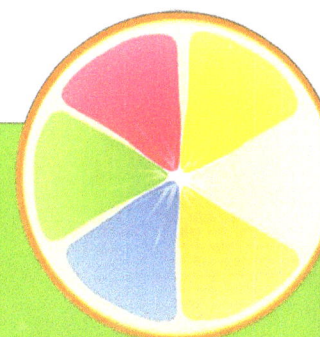

Golden raisins

Raisins are dense in iron. They are a good source of potassium and high in antioxidants.

Easy Way to Incorporate Orange and Yellow Fruits and Vegetables into Your Diet

- Pack an orange or carrot sticks/ baby carrots as a lunch or a snack for work or school day.

- Shredded carrots (grated on a cheese grater) have a great light consistency. Add some lemon juice and golden raisins to make a carrot salad-- a lovely orange and yellow mix. Torn mint or chopped parsley can also be added.

Test your Orange/Yellow HQ with these questions:

1.) What are carotenoids great for the health of?

2.) What mineral do golden raisins have a lot of?

3.) Which root vegetable has more nutrients, sweet potatoes or white potatoes?

info@HueTrition.com
HueTrition.com

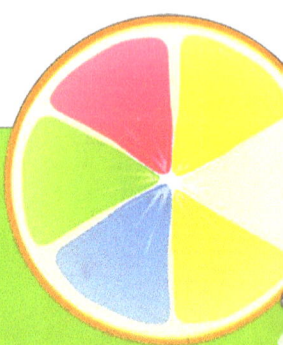

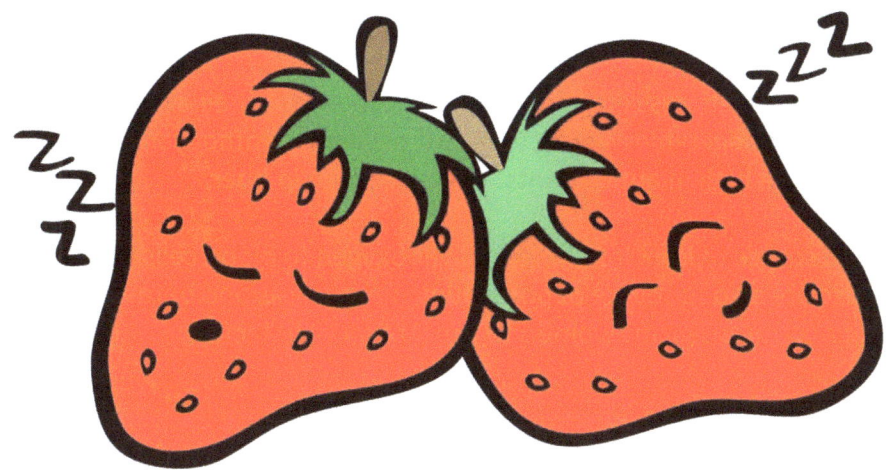

IT'S BEEN A BERRY LONG DAY

CHAPTER 5
Red Fruits and Vegetables

What can we be sure all red fruits and vegetables have in common? Antioxidants. One of the most common in red fruits and vegetables are anthocyanins, which are also responsible for the color. Anthocyanins are a type of flavonoid.

Anthocyanins and flavonoids in general are antioxidants. Anthocyanin is released into the layer of cells that coat the cardiovascular system and provides antioxidant protection from oxidative stress. Anthocyanins protect cells from damage. They may reduce cancer and stroke risk, and heart disease.

Beets, red cabbage, red bell peppers, rhubarb, red potatoes, red onions, radicchio, radishes, tomatoes, cactus pears, tomatoes, cranberries, cherries, red grapes, strawberries, raspberries, red apples, pomegranates, blood oranges, red pears, guava, pink grapefruit, watermelon, cactus pears

info@HueTrition.com
HueTrition.com

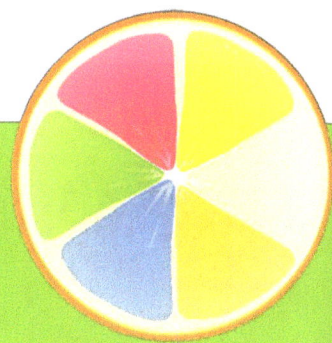

Beets

Ruby red beets are sometimes referred to as "dirt candy" for their sweet flavor.
Beets, like other red vegetables are rich in anthocyanins. Anthocyanins help protect and repair DNA. Beets are high in antioxidants. Beets are high in fiber.

Beets are a good source of iron. Iron helps deliver oxygen to blood cells and is a good energy source. They also are a good source of potassium, manganese, and beta- carotene. Beets are high in folate, great for pregnant women to prevent birth defects.

Red cabbage

Being part of the cruciferous family red cabbage is rich in "indoles", cancer-fighting compounds also found in green cabbage broccoli, brussel sprouts, swiss chard, and kale. Red cabbage has a healthful compound that green vegetables don't. They have what a lot of the fruits and vegetables in this category have- the powerful antioxidants anthocyanins.

Red Chiles

Chili peppers have vitamin C, vitamin B-6, vitamin A, vitamin B-2, copper, calcium, magnesium, phosphorus, and potassium.

Red Bell Peppers

Red bell peppers have up to 3 to 4 times the vitamin C of green bell peppers.

Rhubarb

Rhubarb is a good source of vitamin C, fiber, and calcium.

Red potatoes

They are high in vitamin C and vitamin B6 and significant levels of copper and potassium.

Red onions

Quercetin is found red onions. Onions are a source of calcium, phosphorus, zinc and vitamin C. The purplish tone in red onions is due to anthocyanins.

info@HueTrition.com
HueTrition.com

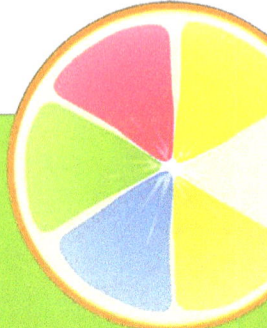

Radicchio

Radicchio is a little bitter in flavor. Radicchio has antioxidant power as high as blueberries or spinach. It can be sautéed or grilled, and drizzled with reduced balsamic vinegar.

Radishes

Radishes are an excellent source of vitamin C. They are a good source of potassium and folic acid.

Tomatoes

Tomatoes have lycopene. Lycopene is responsible for the red pigment in certain foods, and it can also be used as a natural food dye. Lycopene reduces risks of prostate, lung and liver cancers.

Lycopene is absorbed by the body more easily from cooked foods, such as tomato sauce for spaghetti rather than tomatoes. Lycopene is absorbed better with fat, it's fat soluble, so add olive oil to your spaghetti sauce. In fact, the deeper the red color of the fruit or vegetable, the more lycopene it has!

Red grapes

Resveratrol is found in red grapes (as it is in purple grapes), bilberries and cranberries. It is anti-cancer, anti-viral, neuro-protective, anti-aging, and anti-inflammatory. This compound is also found in red wine made from purple or red grapes.

Easy Ways to Incorporate Red Fruits and Vegetables Into Your Diet

Some terrific ideas are to:

- Roast tomatoes, remove skins, and blend. Strain and add stock to make a delicious tomato soup.
- Put tomatoes in salads
- Pack some strawberries or red apples for lunch

info@HueTrition.com
HueTrition.com

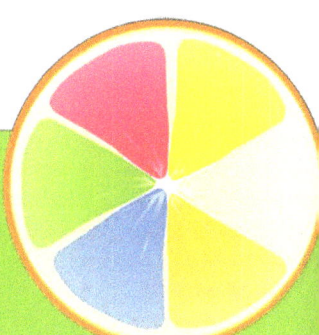

Test your Red HQ with these 4 questions:

1.) What is the major antioxidant found in tomatoes that is also responsible for their red color?

2.) What properties does resveratrol, found in red grapes, have?

3.) What disease do indoles work to prevent?

4.) Which of your body's systems is Vitamin C good for?

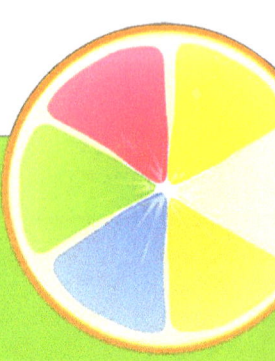

info@HueTrition.com
HueTrition.com

Download HuePets™ 2.0 Today!

For a chance to WIN A Huey Plushie, HuePets lunch/travel bag, and HuePets coloring book

*while supplies last

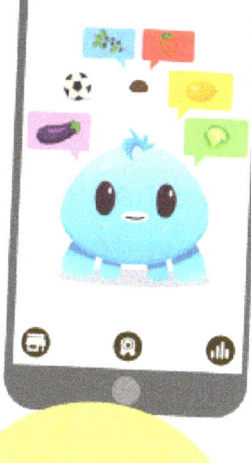

WIN a Huey Plushie Bundle!

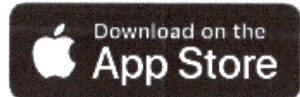 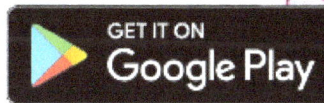

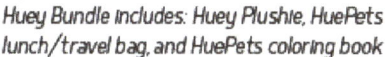

Huey Bundle includes: Huey Plushie, HuePets lunch/travel bag, and HuePets coloring book

If you download and review HuePets app on Google Play or App Store, we will count it as 5 entries towards a chance to with Huey Plushie Bundle! HuePets 2.0 educational promotional materials and collectibles— Huey is a mini companion of healthy choices! Limited quantities for Fall!

If you would like to support our mission and/or get it for your kids or a kid you care about, please reserve yours with this link:
https://huetrition.shop/product/huepets-bundle/

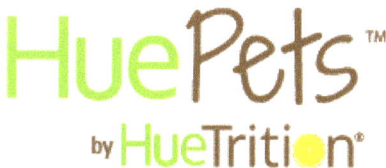

Fun Ways to Get Your Kids to Eat More Fruits and Vegetables

Getting kids to eat fruits and vegetables *can* be a challenge. It doesn't have to be though. HueTrition.com is sharing Fun Ideas that'll turn this parenting challenge into a parenting triumph!

There's an app for that!

Have you heard of the HuePets app? Learn more at www.HuePets.com

With this app, kids scan pictures of the fruits and vegetables they're eating. Then they're able to feed them to a virtual pet-a HuePet that grows and thrives off those healthy foods.

Kids can also play with their HuePet on this colorful, fun app. As the parent, you can set rewards for your child to work towards, track their progress, and receive notifications when they reach their goal.

The best part is that you're able to use technology to encourage your kids to eat their fruits and vegetables. It's a great way to motivate them to make healthy choices.

info@HueTrition.com
HueTrition.com

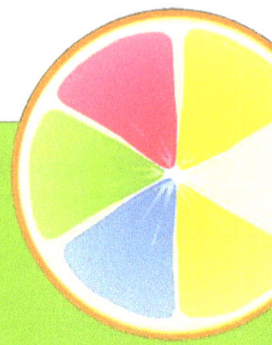

Have you tried out the HuePets app?

Download it today. It's available in both the Apple App Store and on Google Play. HuePets truly is a fun, motivational tool that might just have your kids saying, "More fruits and veggies, please!"

Download the HuePets App at huepets.com

Free Coloring Book

Get your kids even more excited about eating healthy food with this free printable coloring book from HuePets.

Go to huetrition.com to download your copy.

info@HueTrition.com
HueTrition.com

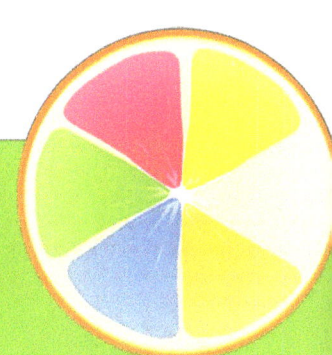

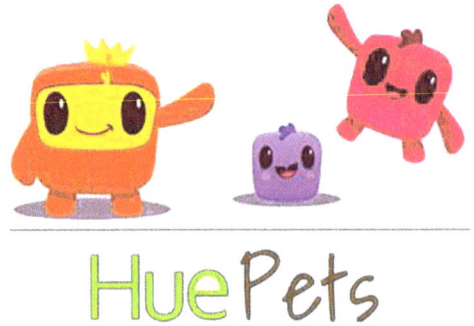

HuePets™ Just for Kids!

Children's Activity Section

What are your answers to these 5 questions?

1.) Have you ever seen a rainbow in the sky? When do rainbows come out?

2.) What is your favorite color of the rainbow? What is a fruit or vegetable that is that color?

3.) Draw your favorite fruit and write or say a sentence about it.

4.) What is your favorite snack that has a colorful fruit or vegetable?

5.) If you were a fruit or vegetable- which one would you be? Why?

info@HueTrition.com
HueTrition.com

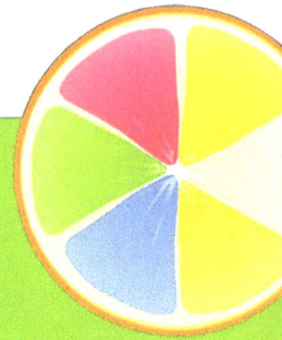

Using our new and innovative program, HuePets™, Eating healthy can be fun!

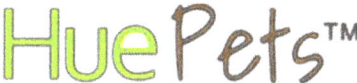

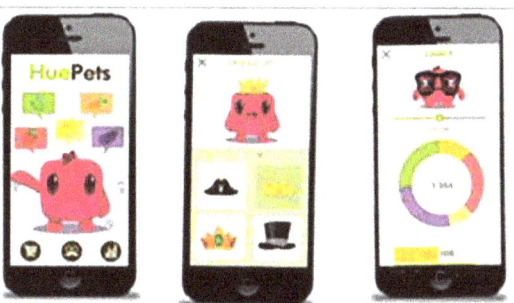

This fun mobile app turns daily healthy eating into a game for young children and their families. Image-Recognition Technology enables kids to "feed" photos of their real-life food to an adorable digital pet, encouraging a well-balanced diet from an early age.

It's so simple to use!

info@HueTrition.com
HueTrition.com

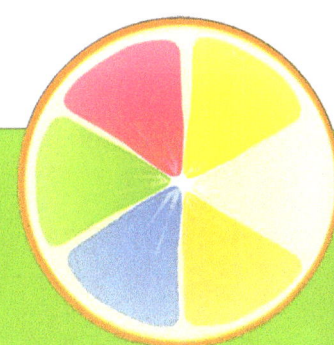

HuePets 2.0, new age program, is the simplest and most fun way to get your kids to eat vegetables!

1. A FREE mobile app that turns daily healthy eating into a game- new characters!
2. The app is tied to a website that allows medical professionals, teachers, family, and friends to view a patients or kids dashboard of colorful choices and even assign rewards!
3. HuePets educational promotional materials and collectibles—including the Huey Bundle: First edition Huey Plushie, HuePets coloring book, and HuePets lunch-bag. To get your Huey Bundle, please visit:

https://huetrition.com/asseenontv/

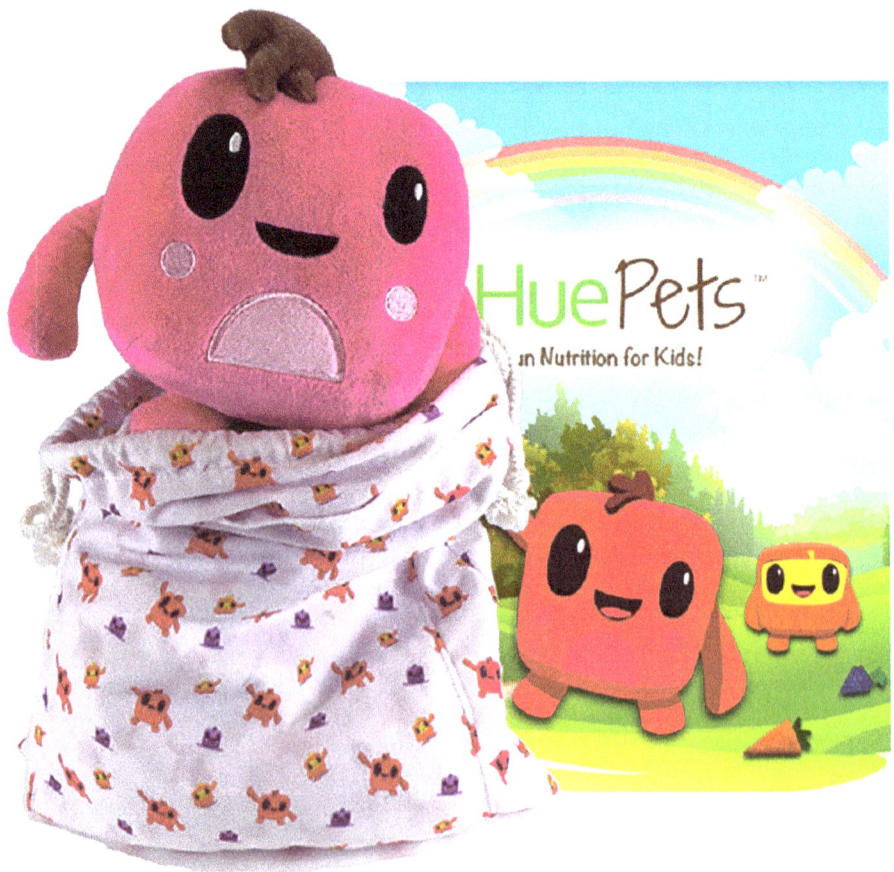

info@HueTrition.com

HueTrition.com

FRUIT AND VEGETABLE JOKES

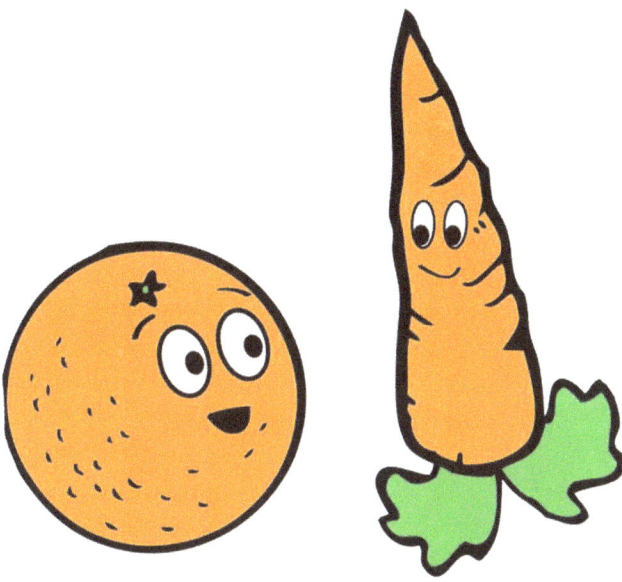

"ORANGE YOU GLAD WE'RE BFF'S?"

Knock, Knock
Who's there?
Banana, Knock, Knock.
Who's there?
Banana, Knock, Knock
Who's there?
Orange
Orange who?
Orange you glad I didn't say "banana"?

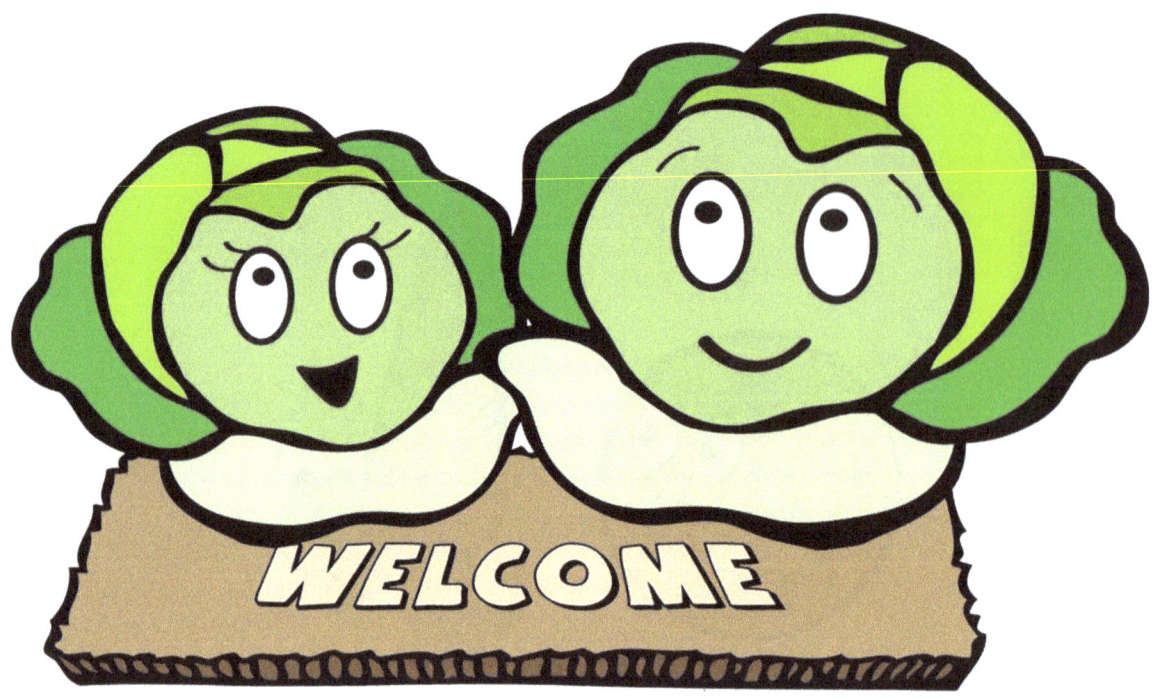

"CAN YOU LETTUCE IN?"

Knock, Knock
Who's there?
Lettuce
Lettuce who?
Lettuce in and you'll find out!

info@HueTrition.com
HueTrition.com

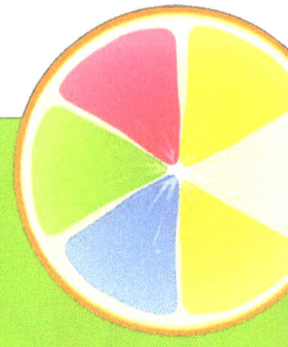

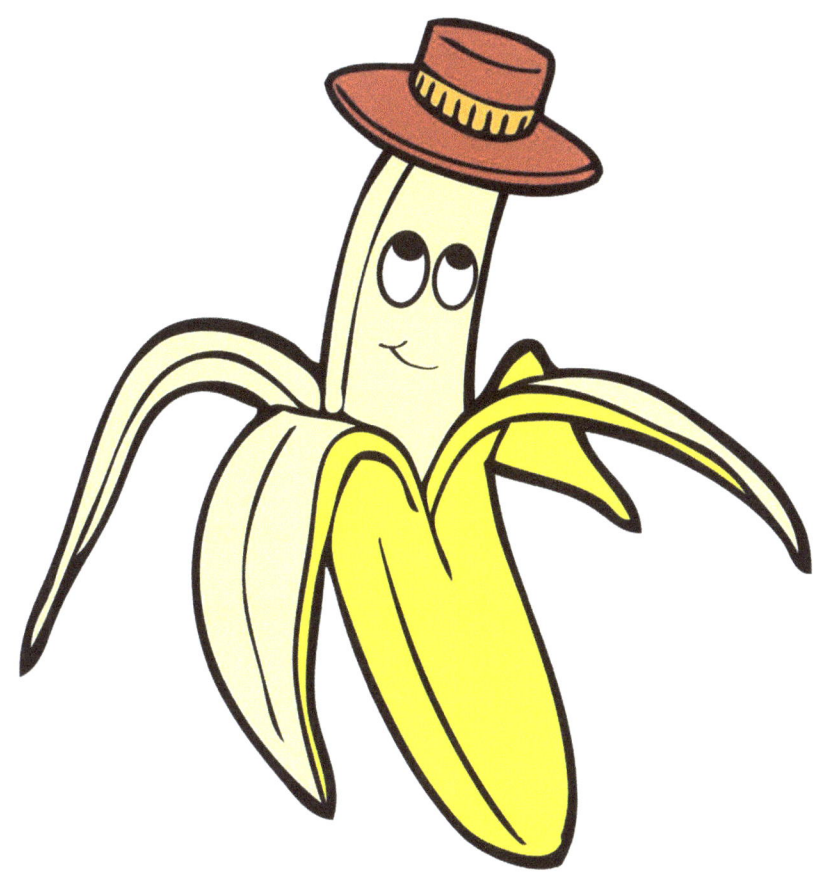

THIS HAT MAKES ME "A-PEELING"

Question: Why did the banana go to the doctor?
Answer: Because it wasn't peeling well.

Question: What is red and blushes? Answer: An embarrassed tomato!

Question: Why is it not a good idea to tell too many secrets in a cornfield?
Answer: There are too many ears!

Question: What kind of vegetable likes to look at animals?
Answer: A zoo-chini!

info@HueTrition.com
HueTrition.com

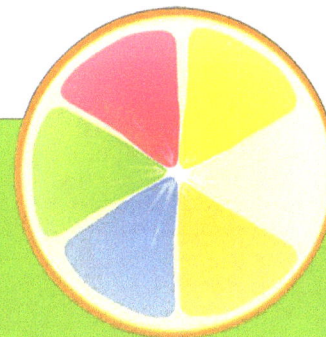

HueKid Poems

Things I wonder when I wonder why
I wonder why…
Fruits are all the colors of a rainbow in the sky
Vegetables too? Oh my!
Oh, the things I wonder when I wonder why….

My tongue is blue.
What did I do?
I ate blueberries.
And look, you did too!

Do you know the answers to the questions below? Test your HQ! Answer these 7 questions:

1.) What one of these choices lists fruits that only *seem like* vegetables?

   a.) radish and celery
   b.) carrot and cucumber
   c.) avocado and tomato
   d.) green peppers and yams

2.) List 5 fruits (one from each color) that are shaped like circles:

   a.)
   b.)
   c.)
   d.)
   e.)

3.) When you bite into a fresh apple, what does it taste like?

   a.) crunchy and juicy
   b.) chewy and salty
   c.) smelly and squishy
   d.) prickly and spicy

info@HueTrition.com
HueTrition.com

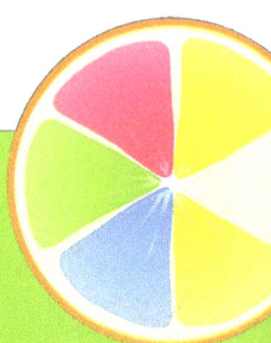

4.) What is a vegetable we see a lot on Halloween?

   a.) pumpkin
   b.) cucumber
   c.) potato
   d.) peach

5.) What vegetable does a bunny like that is also good for kids eyesight?

   a.) turnips
   b.) radishes
   c.) cucumbers
   d.) carrots

6.) What are some vegetables that can taste really spicy?

   a.) carrots and cucumbers
   b.) radish, onion, and chili peppers
   c.) green beans and peas
   d.) broccoli and tomatoes

7.) What are the best ways to grow strong?

   a.) Eat fruits of all different colors
   b.) Eat Vegetables of all different colors
   c.) Play outside or exercise
   d.) All of the above

info@HueTrition.com
HueTrition.com

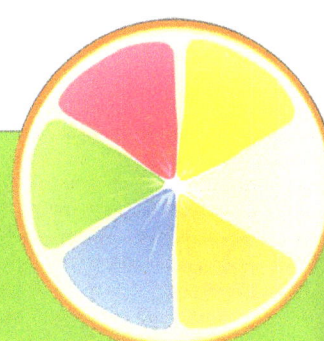

BE A HUEKID: MUNCH YOUR WAY THROUGH THE RAINBOW!!!

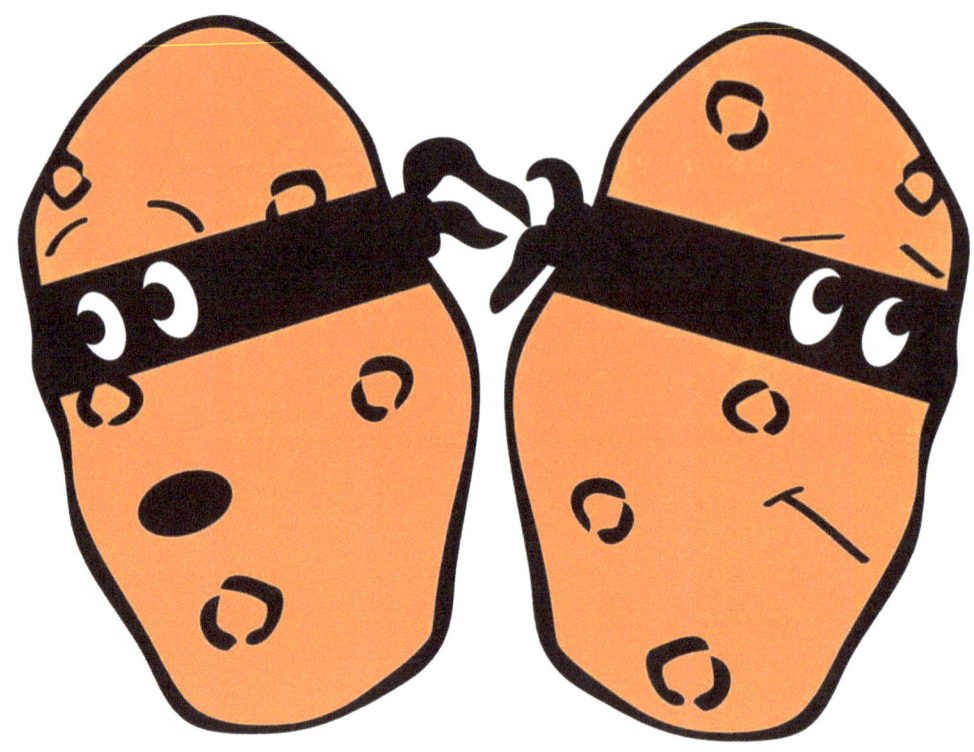

"JUST KEEP YOUR EYES PEELED!"

We like to eat all the different colors of fruits and vegetables at HueTrition. We can group fruits and vegetables into the following color types:

- Blue/purple
- Red
- Yellow/Orange
- White
- Green

info@HueTrition.com
HueTrition.com

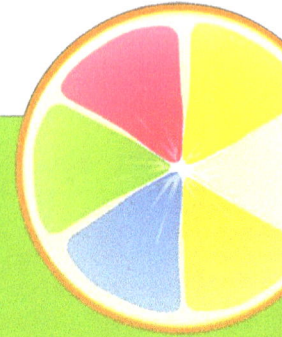

CHAPTER 6
Blue/Purple Fruits and Vegetables

Some things I always wonder are why are blueberries blue? Why are grapes purple?

Grapes and blueberries are purple because of what they are made of. The same compound that gives them their color, gives them their health benefits. Their blue and purple colors are a clue to what nutrients are inside.

Did you know that sometimes you can find purple carrots or blue potatoes? Sometimes farmers grow them and sell them at farmer's markets.

Have you ever been to a farmers market? Farmers markets are where farmers go to sell their fruits and vegetables to people.

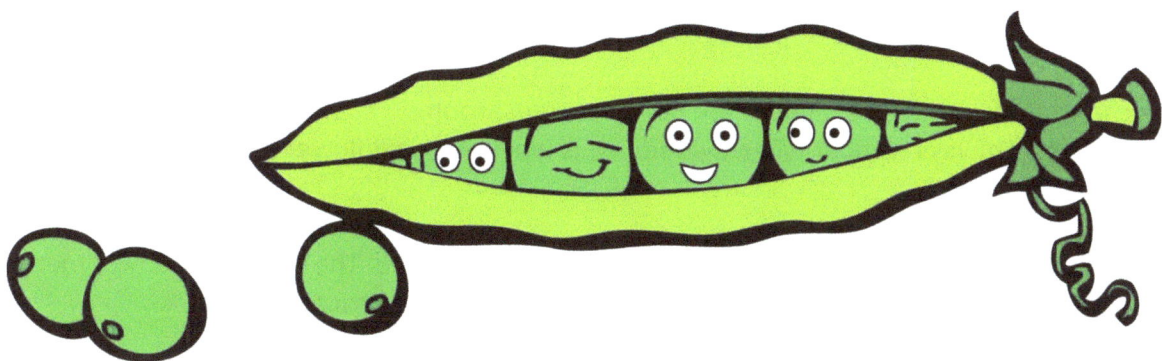

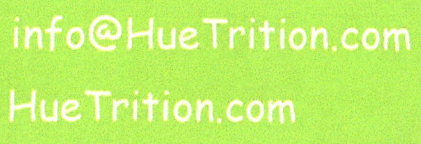

info@HueTrition.com
HueTrition.com

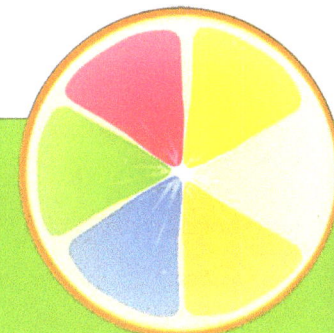

CHAPTER 7
Green Fruits and Vegetables

I'm a lean green string_____.
I'm a round, little, light green sweet_____.

What green fruits grow on trees?
Hmmm, let's see... green apples, limes, pears and kiwis grow from trees!

What green vegetables grow straight from the ground?
Hmmm, let's see.... Celery, broccoli, green beans and peas grow from the ground!

CHAPTER 8
White Fruits and Vegetables

Some white fruits and vegetables are potatoes, mushrooms, cauliflower,
Something I always wonder when I wonder.... is why does cauliflower have the word flower in it? Is it a flower?

Yes, cauliflower is made of flower buds that have not developed. The name cauliflower means "cabbage flower." Did you know that cauliflower is related to broccoli?

info@HueTrition.com
HueTrition.com

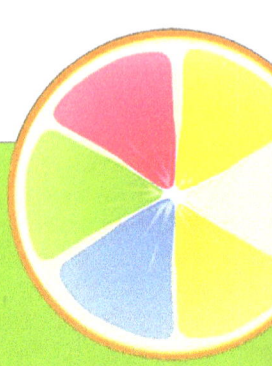

CHAPTER 9
Yellow/Orange Fruits and Vegetables

Something I always wonder when I wonder is....Do monkeys really eat bananas? Why?

I know the answer! Monkeys eat bananas because they are often available in their environment. They also eat them for the same reasons we do- they are sweet and full of potassium for energy!

Some orange fruits and vegetables that are good for growing kids are oranges, carrots, sweet potatoes and more.

Fruits and vegetables, including orange ones, can help our health in different ways. For example, carrots are good for your eyes, and eating oranges helps you to not get sick, and can even help to make our colds shorter.

info@HueTrition.com
HueTrition.com

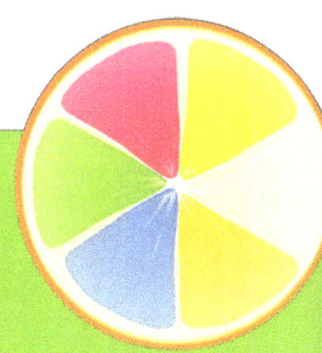

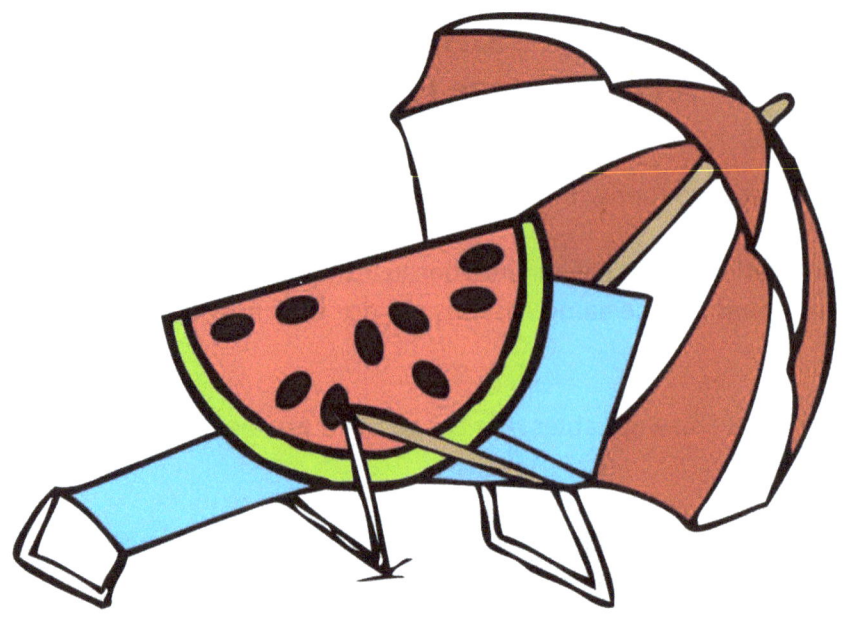

"I'M NOT ACTUALLY A FAN OF WATER."

CHAPTER 10
Red Fruits and Vegetables

Strawberries, cherries, and apples are delicious. Did you ever go strawberry or apple picking? Did you ever see a strawberry or apple growing? Did you ever see anything red growing?

If you've seen an apple growing, you have seen it growing from a tree. Strawberries grow from the ground.

Something I always wonder when I wonder is…. Where does my fruit come from and how does it get to my house? A nice thing to do is visit a garden or a farm. There you can see where the fruit grows before it gets shipped to the store.

info@HueTrition.com
HueTrition.com

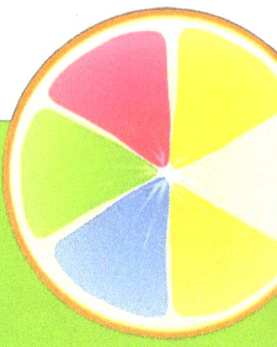

Why is a tomato considered a fruit and not a vegetable? According to science a fruit is the part of the plant that you can eat that comes from the flower, like tomatoes.

That makes me wonder... if fruits come from the flower of the plant, where do vegetables come from?

A vegetable can grow from the leaves of the plant, the stem, or the roots, but not the flower.

Did you ever wonder why fruits are sweet?

Fruits have natural sugars called glucose and fructose. Most red fruits like cherries, strawberries, and apples are the sweet part of the plants they grow from.

Because they are bright and sweet, animals want to eat them. Since seeds are part of the fruit, when animals go to the bathroom, the seeds get left on the ground. More plants with fruits can then grow from these seeds!

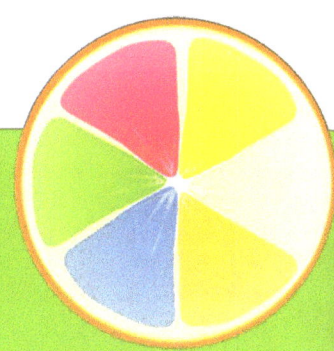

info@HueTrition.com
HueTrition.com

CHAPTER 11
Putting HueTrition to Work

5 Easy Recipes for Adults to Make for Family (1 of Each Color)

Blueberry Pancakes
Serves 4

Ingredients

3-1/2 cups AP flour
1 tablespoon baking powder
1 cup sugar
3 eggs, beaten
1 stick butter
1 cup whole milk
1 cup blueberries
Vegetable oil or butter for cooking

Directions

Mix together the dry ingredients- flour, baking powder, salt, and sugar. Whisk the beaten eggs into the flour mixture. Mix the butter and milk into a bowl, and then whisk into the pancake batter.

Heat a griddle, pan, or skillet with oil on medium heat. Put about 3 or 4 tablespoons of the mixture in the pan to form a circle to make a pancake. Drop 8 blueberries on each pancake. Once bubbles form on the surface of the pancakes, flip and cook the other side until the pancake is cooked through.

Serve with maple syrup and butter.

info@HueTrition.com
HueTrition.com

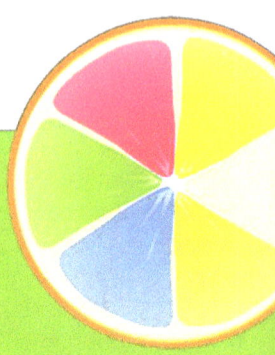

Sweet Yams with Golden Raisins
Serves 4

Ingredients

1 cup golden raisins
3 thinly sliced medium sized sweet potatoes or yams
2 to 3 cups chicken stock or broth

Directions

Cook all ingredients over medium heat at a simmer until yams are tender and raisins are hydrated. Use a potato masher, or a stand mixer to mash or whip the potatoes. Enjoy.

Roasted Broccoli with Garlic and Lemon
Serves 4

Ingredients

2 heads broccoli florets
1 tablespoon olive oil
1 garlic clove, minced
1 teaspoon salt
1/2 teaspoon ground pepper
1/2 lemon, juiced

Directions

Preheat the oven to 400 degrees. Carefully wash broccoli and cut off the ends, leaving the stalks and florets attached. Toss the broccoli spears in olive oil, minced garlic, salt, and pepper. Spread evenly on a baking sheet. Roast for 15 to 20 minutes until the broccoli stems are tender when pierced with a fork. Remove from baking sheet and sprinkle or toss with lemon juice.

For extra color and deliciousness, you can even toss in red bell pepper strips and cherry tomatoes to roast with the broccoli!

info@HueTrition.com
HueTrition.com

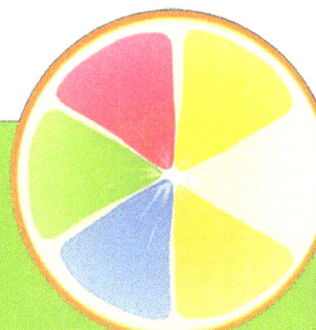

Mashed Cauliflower
Serves 4

Ingredients

1 head cauliflower, cut into small florets
2 tablespoons extra virgin olive oil
Salt and freshly ground black pepper to taste

Directions

Boil a large pot of water with salt. Add cauliflower to boiling water and cook for 10 minutes, until really tender. Reserve ¼ cup water.

Put cauliflower in a food processor or blender and puree with the reserved water and olive oil, adding only a little of the liquid at a time until desired texture is achieved. Add salt and pepper to taste.

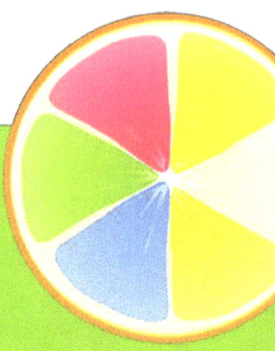

info@HueTrition.com
HueTrition.com

"Tomato" Spaghetti Sauce (with Beets!)

Ingredients

1 can tomato sauce
2 tablespoons tomato paste
4 beets, roasted and peeled, peeled and boiled, or canned
2 cloves garlic, minced
torn basil leaves
1 tablespoon oregano
1 tablespoon sugar or 2 tablespoons grape juice (or red wine), optional
2 tablespoons olive oil
Salt and freshly ground black pepper, to taste

Directions

Mince garlic finely. In a sauté pan, heat olive oil on medium heat. Add garlic and cook for 30 seconds or until golden and fragrant but not browned. Add tomato sauce and tomato paste to the pan. Puree the beets in a blender with a touch of water and add the red puree to the sauce. Sprinkle in oregano and sugar or grape juice (optional)

Stir and cook over medium low heat. Add freshly torn basil and cook for just a couple minutes more. Add to your favorite cooked pasta.

info@HueTrition.com
HueTrition.com

5 Easy Recipes for Kids to Learn to Make (1 of Each Color)

Do you like to cook? If you do, I have some fun recipes for you!

Red Apples with peanut butter and raisin smiley faces
Serves 4

Ingredients

2 red apples
A handful of golden or purple raisins (or mixed)
3 tablespoons creamy peanut butter

Directions

1.) Core the apples and cut in half.
2.) Spread a layer of peanut butter over each apple half.
3.) Make a smile, eyes, and a nose with the raisins (this is similar to making a snow man)

White- Frozen banana pop
Serves 4

Ingredients

4 bananas, peeled
4 popsicle sticks or skewers

Directions

1.) Peel bananas and put onto popsicle sticks or skewers.
2.) Put in a dish in the freezer for 2 hours until frozen through.

info@HueTrition.com
HueTrition.com

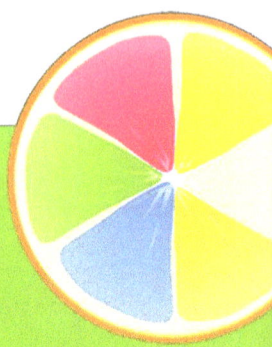

Blue/Purple- Homemade Grape gelatin

Ingredients

1 envelope (1/4 ounce) unflavored gelatin
1/4 cup cold water
1 cup grape juice

Directions

1.) Sprinkle the package of gelatin over cold water in a bowl. Let sit for 5 minutes until soft.
2.) Bring another 1/4 cup of water to boil. Pour this over the gelatin and cold water. Mix.
3.) Stir in the grape juice and refrigerate 1 hour until set.

Yellow/Orange- Carrot sticks or baby carrots with 4 dips

Ingredients
Hummus, store-bought is okay
Creamy salad dressing
Appetizer dips of choice such as guacamole, or chip dip

Directions

1.) Put the baby carrots in a bowl
2.) Arrange dips in small bowls, or spoonfuls of dip around a plate
3.) Do a taste test, which dip is your favorite and which one is your second favorite?

info@HueTrition.com
HueTrition.com

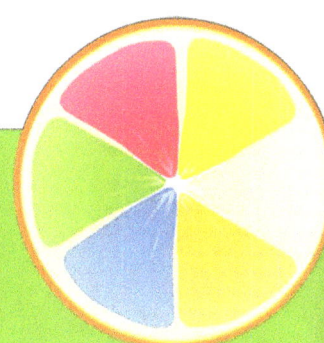

Green Fruit kabobs
Serves 4

Ingredients
4 small skewers
1 green apple, chopped
1 handful green seedless grapes
Honeydew melon, chopped (optional)
1 container vanilla yogurt

Directions

1.) Dollop the vanilla yogurt into bowls for dipping (about 3 tablespoons a bowl)
2.) Skewer the fruit onto small skewers
3.) Dip into yogurt and eat!

HueTrition is about creating a lasting, genuine lifestyle change. Get a jumpstart on improving your eating habits with HueChallenge by going to HueTriton.com to sign-up for our HueNewsletter packed with tips, recipes, and tools. You will notice the positive changes in how your health and how you feel and look!

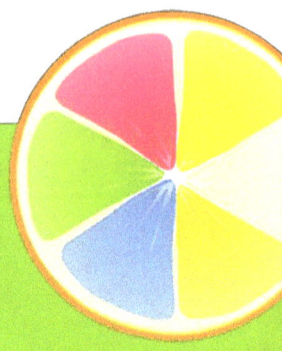

info@HueTrition.com
HueTrition.com

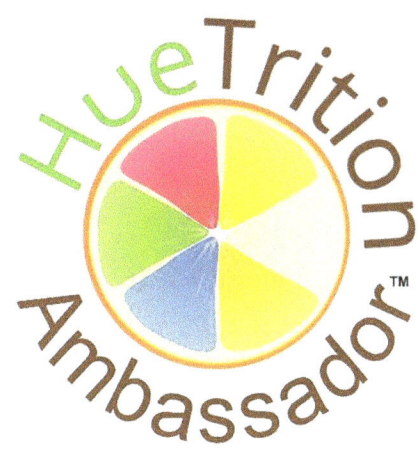

Be a part of the HueMovement™!

You and your kids can be a part of the HueMovement™ by becoming a **HueAmbassador™!**

By becoming a HueAmbassador™, you are pledging to be a part of HueMovement™ which promotes a balanced, active, and healthy lifestyle while encouraging eating colorful fruits and vegetables.

We will provide a HueAmbassador™ Badge to be used on your website and social media!

We will also provide valuable HueTrition™ resources such as our HuePets™ program (app and parent/educator program), educational brochures, our e-book, coloring book, various educational materials, and potential support for live event to help better spread the movement. If you would like information on how you can become a HueAmbassador™, or to receive our resources;

Please contact info@huetrition.com

info@HueTrition.com
HueTrition.com

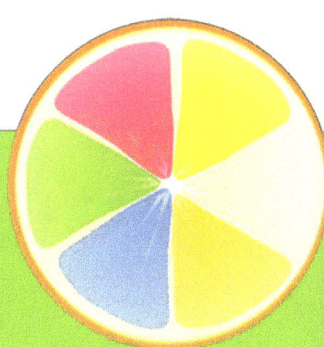

Serving Sizes

At HueTrition we advocate eating a 1 serving of each of the 5 colors a day. You might ask yourself, what is a serving size? Here's a list of the breakdowns for fruits and vegetables and some examples:

1 medium-sized fruit (equal to about 1/2 cup)
1 cup raw leafy vegetables like spinach or lettuce 1/2 cup cooked dry beans or peas
1/4 cup dried fruit
3/4 cup (6 oz.) of 100% fruit or vegetable juice
1/2 cup fresh, frozen, or canned fruit (in 100% juice) or vegetables

Examples include:

Fruits

One banana
One apple
One peach
Six strawberries
Two plums Fifteen grapes
One-half cup of orange, apple, grape or other fruit juice

Vegetables

3/4 cup vegetable juice
Half of a baked sweet potato
One ear of corn
Four slices of an onion
Five cauliflower or broccoli florets
10 baby carrots
One roma tomato
3/4 cup tomato juice

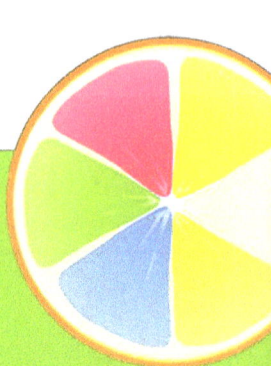

info@HueTrition.com
HueTrition.com

List of Fruits and Vegetables by Color:

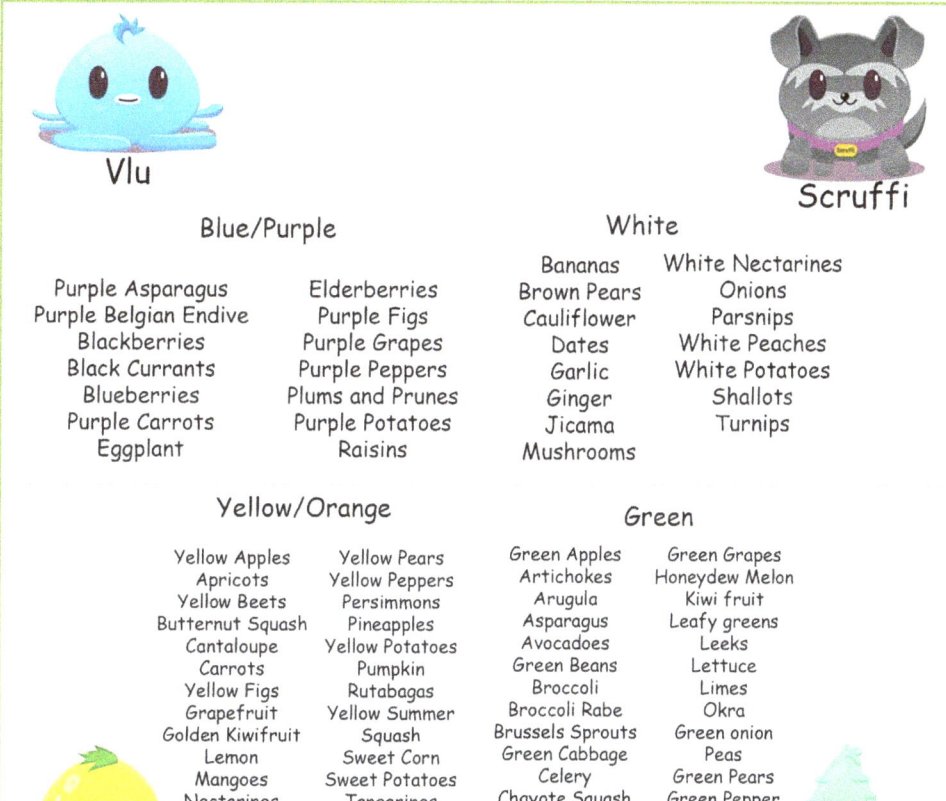

Blue/Purple

- Purple Asparagus
- Purple Belgian Endive
- Blackberries
- Black Currants
- Blueberries
- Purple Carrots
- Eggplant
- Elderberries
- Purple Figs
- Purple Grapes
- Purple Peppers
- Plums and Prunes
- Purple Potatoes
- Raisins

White

- Bananas
- Brown Pears
- Cauliflower
- Dates
- Garlic
- Ginger
- Jicama
- Mushrooms
- White Nectarines
- Onions
- Parsnips
- White Peaches
- White Potatoes
- Shallots
- Turnips

Yellow/Orange

- Yellow Apples
- Apricots
- Yellow Beets
- Butternut Squash
- Cantaloupe
- Carrots
- Yellow Figs
- Grapefruit
- Golden Kiwifruit
- Lemon
- Mangoes
- Nectarines
- Oranges
- Papayas
- Peaches
- Yellow Pears
- Yellow Peppers
- Persimmons
- Pineapples
- Yellow Potatoes
- Pumpkin
- Rutabagas
- Yellow Summer Squash
- Sweet Corn
- Sweet Potatoes
- Tangerines
- Yellow Tomatoes
- Yellow Watermelon
- Yellow Winter Squash

Green

- Green Apples
- Artichokes
- Arugula
- Asparagus
- Avocadoes
- Green Beans
- Broccoli
- Broccoli Rabe
- Brussels Sprouts
- Green Cabbage
- Celery
- Chayote Squash
- Chinese Cabbage
- Napa/Boc Choy
- Cucumbers
- Endive
- Green Grapes
- Honeydew Melon
- Kiwi fruit
- Leafy greens
- Leeks
- Lettuce
- Limes
- Okra
- Green onion
- Peas
- Green Pears
- Green Pepper
- Spinach
- Zucchini

Red

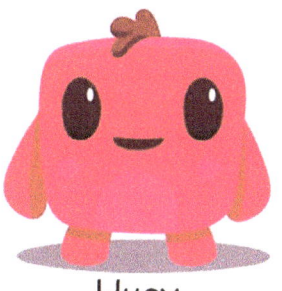

- Red Apples
- Beets
- Blood Oranges
- Red Cabbage
- Cherries
- Cranberries
- Pink/Red Grapefruit
- Red Grapes
- Red Onions
- Red Pears
- Red Peppers
- Pomegranates
- Red Potatoes
- Radicchio
- Radishes
- Raspberries
- Rhubarb
- Strawberries
- Tomatoes
- Watermelon

info@HueTrition.com
HueTrition.com

GLOSSARY

Anthocyanins are the water-soluble hues in a lot of red, purple, or blue fruits or vegetables. Anthocyanins are a type of flavonoid. They are in all sorts of berries and cherries, blood oranges, beets, eggplants, plums and more.

Anthoxanthins are a category of flavonoid color found in plants. They can be white, creamy, or yellow in color. They are found in plant foods such as potatoes and bananas.

Anti-inflammatory is the property of a compound or substance that reduces inflammation. Inflammation in the body can lead to cancers and other diseases.

Antioxidants are substances that protect the body from free radicals. They include substances such as beta-carotene, lycopene, lutein, selenium, vitamins A, C, and E and many phytonutrients.

Beta-Carotene is a yellow, orange, or red hued compound found in vegetables and fruits, like carrots and oranges. Beta-Carotene is a form of vitamin A, and by some estimates it is said to provide nearly 50% of the vitamin A in our diets. Beta-Carotene can be used medicinally to prevent some cancers, heart disease, cataracts and macular degeneration, and many other diseases from schizophrenia to psoriasis.

Blood sugar levels refer to the concentration of the blood glucose level. High levels are called hyperglycemia and low levels can be called hypoglycemia. Certain foods are digested quickly and spike blood sugar leading to an increase, followed by a sharp decrease in energy. Foods with a low glycemic index have slower absorption of sugars in the body, leading to more stable energy.

Flavonoids contribute to beneficial antioxidant activity in the body. They are polyphenolic compounds that are categorized into: flavonols, flavones, flavanones, isoflavones, catechins, anthocyanidins, and chalcones. Many flavonoids are thought to have antiviral, anti-inflammatory, anti-allergic, antioxidant and anti-tumor capabilities or activities.

Free Radicals are molecules made when the body breaks down food, by simply breathing, or is exposed to environmental toxins like cigarette smoke or radiation. They can damage cells and may contribute to heart disease, cancer, and other diseases. As your cells produce energy,

info@HueTrition.com
HueTrition.com

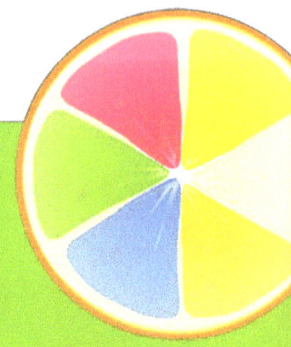

some highly reactive molecules are produced called free radicals. They can cause oxidative damage to proteins, membranes, and genes. They can cause oxidative stress or damage.

Glycemic Index (GI) is the measure of effects of carbohydrates on blood sugar levels. Carbohydrates that digest quickly and release glucose quickly into the bloodstream have a high GI. Carbohydrates that break down more slowly have a low GI and release glucose more slowly and steadily into the blood.

Oxidative Stress or oxidative damage is the result of free radicals. It has been called out as the cause of many diseases. Antioxidants can neutralize free radicals in the body and prevent oxidative stress.

Pectin is a soluble fiber. The pectin from apples, grapes, berries, peaches, currants, and plums is used to make a natural gel for jams or jellies. It is beneficial to health. It can bind to fat and flush it from the body. It can also lower cholesterol levels.

Phenols/ Phenolic acid/ Polyphenols are a group of antioxidant compounds in plants that may reduce the risk of heart disease, cancer, and many other diseases.

Phytonutrients or **phytochemicals** are organic compounds in plants thought to promote health. Unlike fats, proteins, vitamins, and minerals they are not considered essential for life. Phytonutrients include carotenoids, flavonoids, inositol, lignans, isothiocyanates and indoles, phenols, saponins, sulfides, and terpenes.

Quercetin is a flavonoid that occurs in plants, vegetables, grains, fruits, and leaves. Fruits such as cherries, broccoli, pears, grapes and apples contain significant amounts of quercetin.

Resveratrol is an antioxidant that can be found in grape skins, raspberries, cranberries, and blueberries, as well as peanuts. Resveratrol activity has been studied for its possibilities of being anti-aging, fighting memory loss, extending exercise tolerance, and to fight viruses.

info@HueTrition.com
HueTrition.com

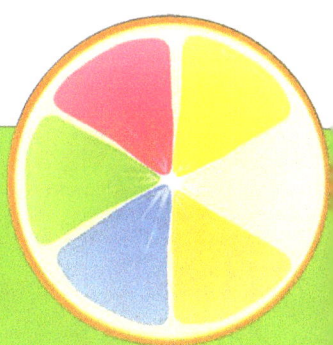

SOURCES

"Raisin." *Wikipedia, the Free Encyclopedia*. Web. 07 Nov. 2011. <http://en.wikipedia.org/wiki/Raisin>.

"Simple Ways to Add Fruits and Vegetables to Your Diet | American Diabetes." *American Diabetes |*. Web. 31 Oct. 2011. <http://www.americandiabetes.com/living- diabetes/diabetes-food-articles/simple-ways-add-fruits-and-vegetables-your-diet>.

The World's Healthiest Foods. Web. 01 Nov. 2011. <http://www.whfoods.com/genpage.php?tname=foodspice>.

"Win Over Picky Eaters . Food & Fitness . PBS Parents | PBS." *PBS: Public Broadcasting Service*. Web. 28 Oct. 2011. <http://www.pbs.org/parents/food-and-fitness/eat- smart/win-over-picky-eaters>.

"Grapes Nutrition Facts and Health Benefits." *Nutrition Facts in the Food You Eat and the Impact on Your Health*. Web. 22 Oct. 2011. <http://www.nutrition-and- you.com/grapes.html>.

Whittemore, Frank. "Nutritional Value Of Red-skin Potatoes | LIVESTRONG.COM." *LIVESTRONG.COM - Lose Weight & Get Fit with Diet, Nutrition & Fitness Tools | LIVESTRONG.COM*. Web. 20 Oct. 2011. <http://www.livestrong.com/article/264105- nutritional-value-of-red-skin-potatoes/>.

"Radishes - Nutrition Information, Health Benefits of Radishes." *Nutrient Information for Whole Foods*. Web. 22 Oct. 2011. <http://www.everynutrient.com/healthbenefitsofradishes.html>.

"Antioxidants and Oxidative Stress." *NetDoctor.co.uk - The UK's Leading Independent Health Website*. Web. 07 Nov. 2011. <http://www.netdoctor.co.uk/focus/nutrition/facts/oxidative_stress/oxidativestress.ht m>.

"Apple Pectin Benefits and Information." *Natural Health Herbal, Vitamin and Nutritional Supplements | NutraSanus*. Web. 07 Nov. 2011. <http://www.nutrasanus.com/apple- pectin.html>.

info@HueTrition.com
HueTrition.com

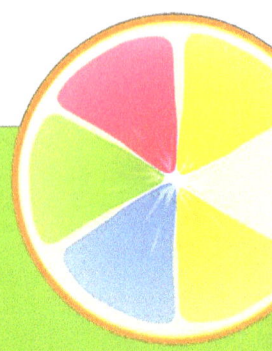

Buhler, PHD, Donald R., and Cristobal Miranda, PHD. "Antioxidant Activities of Flavonoids." *Linus Pauling Institute at Oregon State University*. Web. 07 Nov. 2011. <http://lpi.oregonstate.edu/f-w00/flavonoid.html>.

"MedlinePlus - Health Information from the National Library of Medicine." *National Library of Medicine - National Institutes of Health*. Web. 07 Nov. 2011. <http://www.nlm.nih.gov/medlineplus>.

"Flavonoid." *Wikipedia, the Free Encyclopedia*. Web. 07 Nov. 2011. <http://en.wikipedia.org/wiki/Flavonoid>.

"Anthoxanthin." *Wikipedia, the Free Encyclopedia*. Web. 07 Nov. 2011. <http://en.wikipedia.org/wiki/Anthoxanthin>.

Jegtvig, Shereen. "Serving Sizes for Fruits and Vegetables." *About Nutrition - Healthy Foods, Diet and Weight Loss Advice*. Web. 08 Nov. 2011. <http://nutrition.about.com/od/fruitsandvegetables/f/servingfruit.htm>.

USDA's MyPlate - Home Page. Web. 08 Nov. 2011. <http://www.choosemyplate.gov/>.

info@HueTrition.com
HueTrition.com

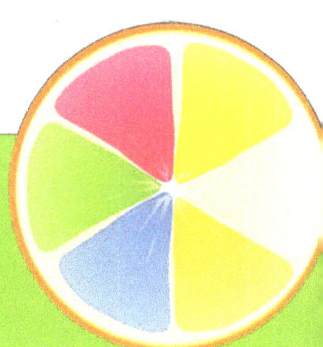

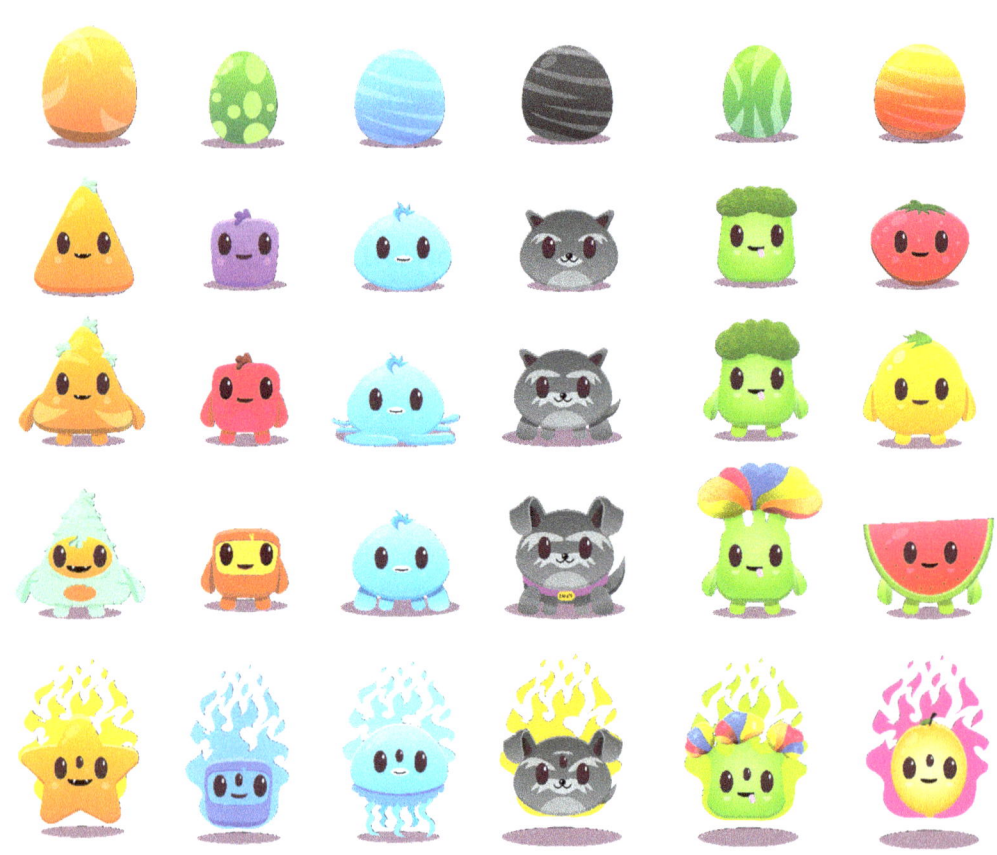

HuePets.com

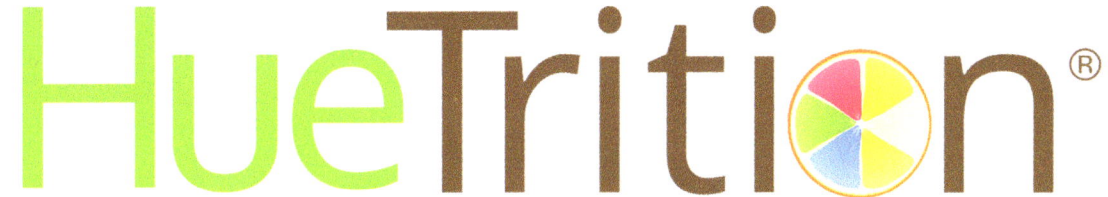

To Learn About Our Mission, please visit:

HueTrition.com

Please follow us on Social Media!

 | | | | |

"A Green Planet has many Colors. Embrace them."

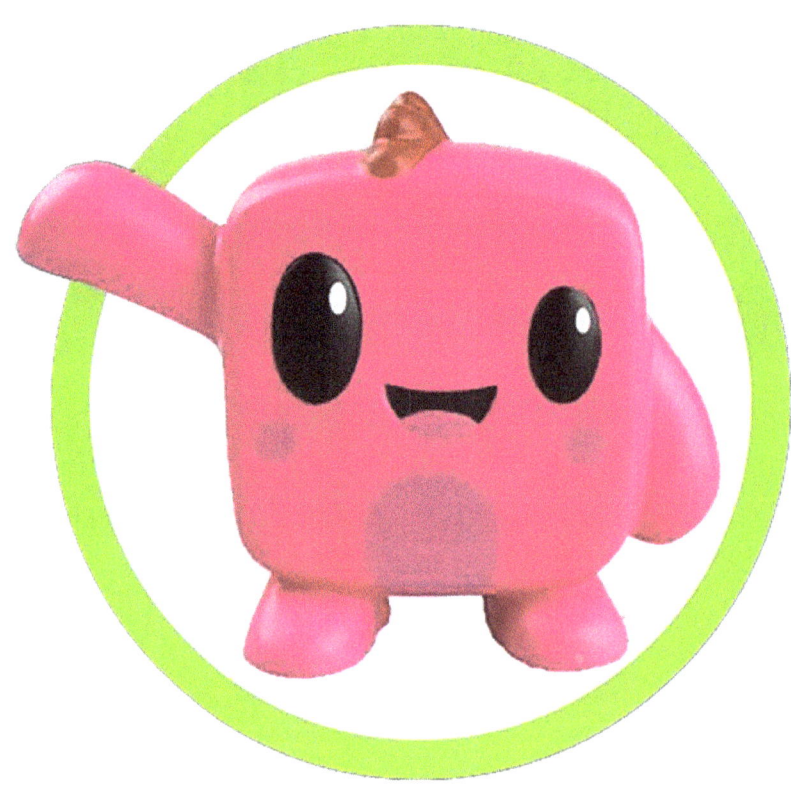

www.ingramcontent.com/pod-product-compliance
Lightning Source LLC
Chambersburg PA
CBHW081203020426
42333CB00020B/2614